Labour Ward Manual

For Churchill Livingstone:

Senior Commissioning Editor: Mary Seager
Development Editor: Catharine Steers
Project Manager: Jane Dingwall/Pat Miller
Design Direction: George Ajayi

Labour Ward Manual

Edited by

David T Y Liu MPhil(BioEng) MB BS DM FRCOG FRANZCOG MBA(OU)
Consultant Obstetrician and Gynaecologist/Clinical Director
Nottingham City Hospital NHS Trust

THIRD EDITION

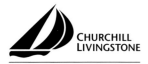

CHURCHILL
LIVINGSTONE

EDINBURGH   LONDON   NEW YORK   OXFORD   PHILADELPHIA   ST LOUIS   SYDNEY   TORONTO   2003

Churchill Livingstone
An imprint of Elsevier Science Limited

First edition 1985
Second edition 1991
Third edition 2003

ISBN 0 443 07394 5

British Library Cataloguing in Publication Data
A catalogue record for this book is available from the British Library

Library of Congress Cataloging in Publication Data
A catalog record for this book is available from the Library of
Congress

Notice
Medical knowledge is constantly changing. Standard safety
precautions must be followed, but as new research and clinical
experience broaden our knowledge, changes in treatment and drug
therapy may become necessary or appropriate. Readers are advised
to check the most current product information provided by the
manufacturer of each drug to be administered to verify the
recommended dose, the method and duration of administration, and
contraindications. It is the responsibility of the practitioner, relying on
experience and knowledge of the patient, to determine dosages and
the best treatment for each individual patient. Neither the Publisher
nor the editor and contributors assumes any liability for any injury
and/or damage to persons or property arising from this publication.
                                                        The Publisher

 your source for books,
journals and multimedia
in the health sciences
www.elsevierhealth.com

The
publisher's
policy is to use
**paper manufactured
from sustainable forests**

Printed in China

Contents

Contributors

Sabaratnam Arulkumaran DCH FRCS FRCOG
FAMS MD PhD HonFACOG FSLOG FSOGC
Professor and Head of Department of Obstetrics
and Gynaecology, St George's Hospital Medical
School, London

Philip Baker DM MRCOG
Professor and Director, Maternal and Fetal
Health Research Care, St Mary's Hospital,
Manchester

Christine Bowman BA MA FRCP
Consultant Physician Genito-urinary Medicine,
Nottingham City Hospital NHS Trust,
Nottingham

Rosemary Buckley BSc RGN RM
Senior Audit Midwife, Nottingham City
Hospital NHS Trust, Nottingham

David A. Curnock MB Bchir FRCP FRCPCH DCH
DObstRCOG
Consultant Paediatrician, Nottingham City
Hospital NHS Trust, Nottingham

Toby Fay MD FRCOG
Consultant Obstetrician, Nottingham City
Hospital NHS Trust, Nottingham

Khaled Ismail MD MRCOG
Clinical Lecturer/Specialist Registrar, Academic
Department of Obstetrics and Gynaecology,
North Staffordshire NHS Trust/Keele
University, City General Hospital, Stoke on Trent

Lucy Kean DM MA MRCOG
Sub-specialist in Maternal-Fetal Medicine,
Nottingham City Hospital NHS Trust,
Nottingham

Mark Kilby MD MBBS MRCOG
Reader and Consultant in Fetal Medicine,
Division of Reproductive and Child Health,
Birmingham Women's Hospital, Edgbaston,
Birmingham

Ronald Lamont BSc DM FRCOG
Consultant Obstetrician and
Gynaecologist/Honorary Reader, Northwick
Park and St Marks NHS Trust, Harrow,
Middlesex

David M. Levy FRCA
Consultant Anaesthetist, Anaesthetics
Directorate, University Hospital NHS Trust,
Queen's Medical Centre, Nottingham

David T. Y. Liu MPhil(BioEng) MB BS DM FRCOG
FRANZCOG MBA(OU)
Consultant Obstetrician and Gynaecologist/
Clinical Director, Nottingham City Hospital
NHS Trust, Nottingham

Pamela Loughna MBBS MD FRCOG MRCGP
Consultant Obstetrician/Honorary Senior
Lecturer, Institute of Reproductive and
Developmental Biology, Faculty of Medicine,
Imperial College of Science, Technology and
Medicine, London (now Nottingham City
Hospital NHS Trust)

Sam Mukhopadhyay MD DMB MRCOG
Department of Obstetrics and Gynaecology,
Norwich and Norfolk Hospital, Norfolk

Alexander Omu FRCOG
Professor and Chairman, Department of
Obstetrics and Gynaecology, Faculty of
Medicine, Kuwait University, Kuwait

Renée Page BSc(Medical Science) MD FRCP
Consultant Endocrinologist, Nottingham City
Hospital NHS Trust, Nottingham

Andrew Parsons LLB
Solicitor of the Supreme Court, Messrs
Radcliffes Le Brasseur, Westminster, London

Charles Rodeck DSc FRCOG FRCPath
Professor and Head of Department, Royal Free
and University College Medical School,
Department of Obstetrics and Gynaecology,
London

Amanda Sullivan PhD BA(Hons) PGDip RGN RM
Consultant Midwife, Nottingham City Hospital
NHS Trust, Nottingham

Pamela M. Thwaites SRN SCN NNEB
Community Midwife, Nottingham

Paul Tomlinson FRCA
Consultant Anaesthetist, Anaesthetic
Directorate, University Hospital NHS Trust,
Nottingham

Martin Whittle MD FRCOG FRCP
Professor and Head of Division of Reproductive
and Child Health, Academic Department of
Obstetrics and Gynaecology, Birmingham
Women's Hospital, Birmingham

George S. H. Yeo MBBS FAMS(Singapore) FRCOG
Chief of Obstetrics, Head & Senior Consultant,
Department of Maternal Fetal Medicine, KK
Women's & Children's Hospital, Singapore

Comment

As the mother of four wonderful children all born at the City Hospital under the careful caring professionalism of Mr Liu, I feel well qualified to recommend this book. I have first hand knowledge of the efficient way in which the labour ward is managed. Giving birth is one of the most moving and memorable times of any woman's life; her confidence comes from the team that supports her and creates calm surroundings for her. It is true to say that those memories will stay with her all her life.

Thank you to Mr Liu and his team for fulfilling all those needs.

Emma Rutland
Duchess of Rutland

Preface

Since the last edition of the *Labour Ward Manual* was published there have been significant changes in the emphasis of care for mothers in labour. Although the principles of operative procedures have altered little, an increasing evidence base from research is determining contemporary practice. Changes reflected in national publications from the Department of Health and Royal Colleges such as *Changing Childbirth* (Changing Childbirth: Report of the Expert Maternity Group EMG HMSO, London 1993), *A First Class Service: Quality in the New NHS* (DoH 1998) and modernisation of the NHS (*The New NHS: Modern Dependable*, DoH 1997) place the mother as central to process of care. Furthermore they emphasize the devolvement of uncomplicated pregnancies to midwives and general practitioners whilst obstetricians deploy their specialist skills to the increasing numbers of complex situations presenting to the labour ward. To address the mother's right to expect flexibility of choice and confidence through continuity of care, obstetricians, midwives, neonatologists, anaesthetists and, as necessary, specialists from other disciplines, must function as a team. It is no longer appropriate simply to dispense care. The offer of choice determines the need for a process of negotiation. Following an informed discussion of options as well as expected consequences and outcomes, agreement can be reached on the way forward.

Consent to accept care encompasses an understanding of the available choices. The negotiated outcome incorporates the ingredients of informed choice, safety, dignity and practice, supported by well-structured research.

The editor welcomes these progressive changes within obstetric practice. The ethos of these changes is also the driver in the restructuring of this text. An international team of specialists have been invited to participate as authors. Whether they contributed totally to the chapter or as mentors their main function was to ensure that the contributions are both contemporary and representative. The aim of *Labour Ward Manual* is to ensure that all women receive optimum care at this important time, thus safeguarding the health of the next generation.

Acknowledgements

This book remains dedicated to all those mothers who have taught us so much about how we can look after mothers even better in the future. The continuing efforts of health providers in their search to improve care are not forgotten. I am grateful for the support of my contributors who share the vision of the need for such a text. My thanks to Anne Whitchurch who coordinated production of the text. My wife Pamela and daughter Natasha receive my thanks for their sacrifice of quality time as a family.

Attitudes and conduct

D. Liu

Childbirth is a physiological function. It is natural that mothers should want to perform this function in the way that they consider most appropriate. Individual preconceived ideas, the media and social and cultural background all contribute in varying degrees to the expectations of the mother in labour. Safety of the mother and fetus or newborn must be the prime objective. However, the birth of a baby should also be remembered as a happy and enriching experience. Labour can only be deemed to have been successfully conducted when these ideals are satisfied.

Attendant medical personnel may have views of their own about the conduct of labour. However, the outcome is unlikely to be considered a success unless medical staff feel they have achieved good rapport with the parturient mothers and conducted the labour to enhance the ideals discussed above. The following guidelines may benefit those who have not appreciated the importance of correct attitudes and conduct as salient measures of proper labour ward management:

- A congenial atmosphere should be maintained to emphasize the concept that labour and delivery are not illnesses. This should not lead us to believe that a degree of professionalism is not respected by the mother or attendant partners. Anxiety is associated with childbirth. Modesty is not automatically relinquished merely because the mother is in labour. Decorum and suitable attire enhance this rapport.

- The shift system for staffing means it is seldom possible for the same medical team to attend for the whole course of labour, although supervision remains the prerogative of the obstetrician in charge. All attendants should have a thorough knowledge of the mother's history and preferences. This will avoid inadvertent comments which prejudice rapport and undermine confidence.
- Modern technology is introduced into the labour ward to enhance the safety of the mother and fetus. When the reasons for their use and the value of their application are explained, then these instruments and special equipment will be viewed by parents as ancillary aids rather than an intrusion. For example, showing the mother and her partner the pattern of some basic fetal heart rate recordings can invite a sense of additional involvement and commitment.
- For a mother with her own preferences for the conduct of labour, ascertain the type of antenatal preparation she has had. Within reason support the concepts and practices she expects. Introduction of alternative practices or procedures at this late stage can confuse, with the resultant loss of confidence. Special preferences which may endanger the mother and fetus should be fully discussed, preferably during the antenatal period, so that risk can be explained and minimized. Flexibility in the attitude of the attendant staff is all important, but it is an indictment against our training and values if we jeopardize the welfare of our charges by subscribing without comment to fashionable idiosyncrasies which we believe may put them at risk of possible medical hazards.
- Husbands or partners are encouraged to stay with mothers throughout labour. Demanding or aggressive behaviour on their part may reflect feelings of helplessness in the perceived situation or guilt because they have subjected their partners to the traumas of childbirth. Ensure mothers are comfortable and that if needed there is ready access to analgesia. Ask after the mother's comfort when her partner is present so that he can be verbally reassured by her. If mothers are obviously over-reacting, explain in the presence of the partner that such behaviour is not conducive to an atmosphere of calm for the birth of their baby. This direct approach reinforces communication between the partners to benefit all concerned.
- Husbands or partners are there to provide support and encourage the ethos of participation by both in the birth of their offspring. This role must be emphasized during operative procedures when a reassuring voice or quiet hand clasp can assist maternal relaxation and control.
- Caesarean section performed under regional anaesthesia may be better accepted if the partner attends to support the mother. There is no justification for the partner's presence if general anaesthesia is used. Minors should not attend labours. Their mothers' natural reactions may be misconstrued and may frighten or create anxiety.
- Tact is all important when dealing with mothers whose expectations are not realized. Mothers who approach labour convinced that all things natural are beneficial may be disappointed. Nature is often cruel and capricious and has not endowed all mothers with the means to easy childbirth. A mother's realization that she is not one of Nature's fortunates can come as an unpleasant surprise. Full explanation helps to dispel some of the feelings of guilt and failure when an assisted delivery is anticipated.
- Mothers who are used to positions of responsibility in society may have difficulty in accepting advice or the 'dictates' of labour ward staff whom they may consider more junior. Rapport and confidence are enhanced if these mothers can observe the efficiency and obstetric training exhibited by their attendants.
- A normal obstetric situation can develop rapidly into an emergency. Anticipation through thorough knowledge of the mother's history, and an appreciation by parents of the significance of that history are important. Equally important is knowledge of the correct procedures to be followed when an emergency arises. Regular drills to familiarize all staff with

emergency procedures are essential. A professional, calm approach reduces anxiety and psychological stress.

All of us who attend labouring mothers must learn to appreciate the limitations of our individual expertise and that of the 'system' in which we work. If we maintain the welfare of the mother and fetus as our prime objective, then there should be no reluctance to seek help from more experienced colleagues when required.

Labour is a reminder of Nature's insistence on survival of the fittest. The role of the obstetric team should be to allow what is physiological to continue, but to intervene where appropriate to counter Nature's indiscretions.

Expectations are, however, exceptionally high and when these are not realized the trend is ready resort to legal redress. The challenge is to provide the highest quality of service within the constraints of both fiscal and human resources. Safe delivery for mother and baby becomes a fundamental expected right whilst quality is measured in terms of satisfaction and the softer paraphernalia around the delivery process. This is best achieved by what I describe as negotiated care, when the informed recipient (mother) and providers (medical carers) enter into a dialogue to determine within the boundaries of risk the acceptable option for all. Expectations are underlined at the outset leaving medical carers to focus effort on the process and incorporate issues for quality.

Some mothers will have special requirements. Guidelines for these are set out in Box 1.1.

Box 1.1   Guideline for mothers with special requirements

High expectations and intolerance of any complication mean that mothers may seek legal redress whenever the outcome is unexpected or untoward. Special requirements or wishes to dictate management must be fully discussed, risk and likely outcome explained and these exchanges are then carefully documented. Verbal consent for special procedures such as induction of labour should be notated. Mothers' signatures are required for surgical procedures such as caesarean section or sterilizations. Additional considerations are:

- Mothers are encouraged to indicate their requirements by 'birth plans'. Discuss their contents and ability to comply before the onset of labour.
- Find out reasons behind their requests, for example social and cultural needs or anxiety after previous obstetric experience. Detailed explanation and reassurance may suffice to correct misconceptions.
- Communication is all important. Inadequate communication is the basis of many legal proceedings. Avoid unprofessional loose remarks.
- If the mother's request is difficult to accept discuss care with a colleague or legal representative, if negotiation cannot achieve a compromise.

Informed consent
Mothers' rights and wishes must be a priority. Current guidelines include:

- Medical personnel must be aware of the legal and ethical issues for consent.

- The person obtaining consent must understand the complexity of the request and be able to provide explanations and answer related questions. This includes purpose of request, diagnosis, treatment options, benefits and side effects.
- Consent can be verbal, written or implied. Consent is essential except in emergencies. A mother must understand the implications of consent, her options, her right to refuse and be afforded time for full discussion and consideration.
- Discuss refusal fully to ensure it is not based on misunderstanding or inadequate information. The informed competent mother is entitled to refuse consent.
- If a competent mother refuses consent, she must be asked to sign a disclaimer releasing the doctor or hospital from responsibility. Notify relevant authorities.
- Document discussions.
- A competent minor (under 16 years of age) can give consent for examination or treatment. The courts in England, Wales and Northern Ireland can challenge a minor if essential treatment in her best interest is refused. Parents or the courts can provide consent on behalf of a mother who lacks capacity to consent. No one can give consent on behalf of another competent adult.
- Mothers unable to provide consent (sedated or unconscious) or mothers from certain cultural or religious backgrounds will need consent by parents, guardians or through special arrangements.
- In emergencies the course of action will be dictated by whatever is in the mother's best interest.

2

Legal considerations

A. Parsons

Litigation as a result of medical treatment is increasing. This chapter provides guidance on some of the most common issues likely to arise in the labour ward. However, it is only a brief summary of the local law and in cases of any doubt legal advice must be obtained.

CONSENT

General principles

A patient has the right under common law to give or withhold consent to medical examination or treatment. The courts have ruled that a mentally competent person has an absolute right to refuse to consent to medical treatment for any reason, rational or irrational, or for no reason at all, even where the decision may lead to the patient's own death. No one else (even next of kin) can consent on behalf of an adult patient (whether competent or not). It is a widely held misconception that families can consent on behalf of patients – *they can not*. Different types of consent are outlined in Box 2.1.

Box 2.1 Types of consent

- Implied: Consent not discussed but implied by action. Example is offering arm for venepuncture.
- Verbal: Consent is sought and verbal permission for procedure is obtained. Documentation of this is advised.
- Written: Documentation must be obtained and witnessed if procedure or treatment carries risks or produces side effects.

Obstetric cases

A woman who is mentally competent to make a treatment decision may choose not to have medical intervention, notwithstanding the risk to her health and even though the consequences may be the death or serious handicap of the child she bears, or her own death. It is the patient's right to make such a decision and the medical staff have no power to override this. Furthermore, in such cases the court does not have jurisdiction to declare medical intervention lawful.

Special types of patient

Children (i.e. under 18) Those over 16 can consent to treatment on their own behalf. For those under 16, the person(s) with parental responsibility has the power to make treatment choices for the child, unless the child is 'Gillick competent' in which case the child can consent. The wellbeing of the child is paramount. Application may be made to the court (a Specific Issue Order) to provide legal sanction for a specific action where doubt or dispute arises.

Psychiatric patients Patients with mental illness or disability have the same rights as other patients. Mental illness (even detention under the Mental Health Act) does not of itself render them incompetent to make treatment choices unless it is so severe as to mean that they are unable to make a treatment choice and are thus incompetent (see below). However, patients detained under the Mental Health Act can be treated without consent under the direction of their resident medical officer (RMO) if the treatment is for their mental disorder (section 63 Mental Health Act).

Jehovah's Witnesses Such patients absolutely refuse the transfusion of blood and blood products even where life is put at risk. Alternative treatment should be considered. It is essential to establish the views held by each Jehovah's Witness patient as some transfusion treatments may be acceptable (such as blood salvage techniques, haemodilution, haemodialysis, cardiopulmonary bypass, albumin, immunoglobulin and clotting factors). To administer blood in the face of refusal may be unlawful. Mentally competent adult patients are entitled to make such a refusal. This may be by advance directive (which may be oral or written). Treatment of the children of Jehovah's Witnesses may require application to the court for an Order.

Mental competence

In determining if a patient is mentally competent, and therefore whether she has capacity to consent to or to refuse treatment, the patient must be assessed as being able to:

- understand and retain the treatment information
- believe it and
- weigh it in the balance to make a choice.

Only if the patient can do all this is she capable of consenting. This test relates to the patient's *ability* to make a decision but is not concerned with the rationality of it – a capable patient is entitled to make a wholly irrational decision.

Advance directives

Advance directives (also known as living wills) are decisions made whilst a person has the necessary mental capacity intended to give effect to wishes as to how treatment or care should be provided in the event they lose capacity.

Advance directives are recognized by English law. They are potentially valid instructions as to which medical treatment that person would or would not be prepared to accept if the capacity to decide is subsequently lost. However, clinicians are not legally bound to provide treatment if it conflicts with their professional judgment about the most appropriate treatment. Nevertheless the patient's wishes should be taken into account in deciding the appropriate course of action. Advance directives cannot authorize a doctor to do anything which is illegal. They may express preferences between treatment options or list an individual's values as a basis for others to reach decisions. They can be written or oral.

Healthcare proxies (i.e. the purported delegation to a third party of the right to make a decision to consent to or refuse medical treatment) are not recognized currently in English law.

Treating without consent

Only if the patient is *not* mentally competent can treatment proceed without consent, in which case the following must also apply:

1. The proposed treatment must be necessary to save the patient's life or prevent deterioration in her physical or mental health.
2. The proposed treatment must be in the patient's best interests (N.B. the best interests of the fetus – save to the extent that delivery of a healthy child is in the mother's best interests – do not form part of this test).
3. The treatment must be such as would be accepted as appropriate by a responsible body of medical opinion.

Informed consent

Patients are entitled to receive sufficient information, in a way that they can understand, about proposed treatments, possible alternatives and any significant risks (which may be special in kind or magnitude or special to the patient), so they can make a balanced judgment. Box 2.2 lists the essential features of informed consent.

Box 2.2   Essentials for informed consent

- Document discussions and treatments in detail, particularly when consent is not available or is refused.
- Give information in language which is sensitive and at an appropriate level for easy understanding. Allow time for questions and reflection.
- Information must be balanced and in adequate detail to allow meaningful choice of options.
- Consent must be obtained by the person who will perform or is able to perform the procedure. The person or team performing the procedure must be disclosed.
- Separate or additional consent must be obtained for further procedures – unless treatment is immediately necessary in the patient's best interests when consent cannot be obtained.
- Where training is involved the level of experience and supervision must be indicated.

Applications to the court to authorize medical treatment

If the patient's competence is unclear, the court can be asked to consider this and if it finds that the patient is incompetent it can declare that a proposed treatment is lawful, even if the patient does not consent. Such declarations should be sought before treatment and can be obtained urgently at short notice.

Guidelines for court applications

1. Competent adult patients can refuse treatment.
2. Such a refusal should be recorded in writing by the patient or, if the patient refuses to do so, this should be entered and countersigned in the medical records.
3. If the patient is definitely mentally incompetent, she should be treated in accordance with her best interests.
4. Treat in accordance with any advance directive – if the reliability of this is in doubt, apply to court.
5. Identify concerns over capacity early (e.g. at antenatal clinics).
6. Obtain a psychiatric opinion on mental capacity.
7. Ensure that the patient has legal representation (if patient is unable to instruct solicitors, contact The Official Solicitor, tel: 0207 936 6000).
8. Take account of the following criteria:
   a. Every person is presumed to have capacity to consent to or refuse medical treatment unless and until this presumption is rebutted.
   b. A competent woman who has sufficient capacity to decide can choose not to have medical intervention even though the consequence might be death or serious handicap of the fetus, or her own death.
   c. The graver the consequences of the decision the commensurately greater the level of competence required to take the decision.

d. A patient can lack capacity if some impairment or disturbance of mental functioning renders the person unable to make a decision whether to consent to or to refuse treatment. This might include temporary factors such as confusion, shock, fatigue, pain or drugs which might erode capacity. However, clinicians must be satisfied that such factors are operating to such a degree.

e. Panic induced by fear might paralyse the will and thus destroy the capacity to make a decision.

SURROGACY

Surrogacy is an arrangement made before conception for a mother to hand over her child to another person. The following features of surrogacy should be understood.

- Surrogate agreements do not affect the child's legal parentage – therefore the birth mother and her partner remain parents until the genetic parents obtain a parental responsibility or Adoption Order from the court.
- A surrogacy arrangement is not illegal itself. The mother can lawfully accept payment of her expenses.
- It is not unlawful for medical staff to assist in the delivery of a child subject to a surrogacy arrangement.
- Consent to treatment for the surrogate mother remains her right and she retains all such rights in respect of the fetus/child (i.e. this is not a right of the genetic parents). Genetic parents can only obtain a Parental Responsibility Order 6 weeks after birth. Until this time, parental responsibility remains with the birth parents. Beware the possibility of breaching the birth mother's medical confidentiality.
- Surrogacy arrangements are not enforceable contracts – if the birth mother changes her mind and wishes to keep the baby she is entitled to do so.
- The birth certificate will contain the name of the birth mother, not the genetic mother.

TERMINATION OF PREGNANCY (TOP)

Termination of pregnancy may only be undertaken by a registered medical practitioner in accordance with the provisions of Section 1 of the Abortion Act 1967. Otherwise any termination will be unlawful.

The Abortion Act requires:

1. Two medical practitioners must agree that:
   a. the pregnancy does not exceed 24 weeks and continuance would involve risk, greater than if it were terminated, of injury to the physical or mental health of the mother or existing children; or
   b. termination is necessary to prevent grave permanent injury to the physical or mental health of the woman; or
   c. continuance of the pregnancy would involve risk to the life of the pregnant woman greater than if the pregnancy were terminated; or
   d. there is a substantial risk that if the child were born it would suffer from such physical or mental abnormalities as to be seriously handicapped.
2. In determining a or b account may be taken of the woman's actual or foreseeable environment.
3. TOP must be carried out in an NHS hospital or a place approved for terminations by the Secretary of State.
4. The requirement for the opinion of two registered medical practitioners and for TOP to take place in a hospital need not be met if the termination is immediately necessary to save the life or prevent grave permanent injury to the physical or mental health of the woman.
5. Notification of TOP is required to the Chief Medical Officer at the Department of Health.
6. Staff may not be compelled to take part in TOP and may exercise a conscientious objection to participation in such treatment – save that this exception does not affect any duty to participate in treatment necessary to save the life or to prevent grave permanent

injury to the physical or mental health of a woman.

7. Anything done to procure a miscarriage is unlawful unless authorized by the Abortion Act provisions referred to above.
8. Assisting in suspected illegal abortion can constitute a criminal offence as can procuring, administering or using drugs or instruments otherwise to procure an abortion.

CONFIDENTIALITY

Patient information may not be used for a different purpose or passed to anyone else without the consent of the patient. Patient information means all personal information held in whatever form. It includes medical details and a patient's name and address, financial and domestic circumstances, etc. Patients should be informed of the uses to which information about them may be put.

When confidential information may be passed on

Information may be passed to someone else:

1. Where the patient consents for a particular purpose
2. Where required on a 'need to know' basis if:
   a. The recipient requires the information because of concern with the patient's care and treatment; or
   b. Use of the information can be justified for improving quality of care, public health, coordinating care with other agencies, effective healthcare administration, or teaching; or
   c. As required by legislation or court order; or
   d. Where this can be justified to protect the public to help prevent, detect or prosecute serious crime (e.g. murder, rape, kidnapping, sexual offences, firearms offences, causing death, or making a threat which could cause serious interference with the security of the state, public order, the administration of justice, injury or serious financial loss).

REGISTRATION OF BIRTHS AND STILLBIRTHS

It is the duty of the father or mother to notify the registrar for the sub-district in which the birth takes place within 42 days. If the father or mother are unable to do this the duty falls on the hospital authority in which the child is born.

For stillborn births, the information to be provided to the registrar is a written certificate that the child was not born alive which must be signed by the registered practitioner or midwife in attendance at the birth or who has examined the body. A stillborn child is one born after 24 weeks of pregnancy who did not breathe after birth.

If an abandoned baby is found the obligation to notify the registrar falls on the person finding the child.

For adopted children, the obligation falls on the natural mother and father.

All births (in hospital or at home) must be notified by a doctor or midwife attending at the birth to the District Medical Officer within 36 hours.

NEGLIGENCE

Medical staff owe patients a duty of care. The standard of care is to act in accordance with practice that would be accepted by a responsible body of similar practitioners.

There is no breach of the standard of care if:

1. you act in accordance with practice accepted by your peers and this was appropriate in this case
2. there is no accepted body of opinion for this situation but what you did was reasonable in all the circumstances
3. you did not follow accepted practice but what you did was reasonable in the circumstances.

Table 2.1 highlights some common situations that may lead to litigation and suggests some actions that could help to avoid problems.

Table 2.1 Common situations leading to litigation – and how to avoid them

Complaint	Prevention
Patient did not consent	Ensure a patient has full information and consents to any treatment
Shoulder dystocia	Ensure senior staff are involved in delivery and carry out drill procedures
Cardiotocograph tracing shows ominous fetal heart rate patterns	Call for prompt medical assistance
Delay in proceeding to caesarean section in an emergency	Ensure all staff are aware of warning signs for the need to proceed to operative delivery and put in place necessary protocols to ensure this is achieved quickly (decision to delivery in 30 minutes)
Fetus delivered too early 'by dates'	Double check dates at each antenatal appointment
Damage to the perineum	Experienced staff to follow established protocols

MEDICAL RECORDS

Clear, detailed medical records enable communication amongst the clinical team. As such they are an important part of ensuring the quality of patient care. They also provide the best defence for staff when matters go wrong. Full and detailed notes should be made in all cases and clearly signed by the member of staff making them. A failure to do so may strengthen a claim for compensation, or the fact that notes are incomplete can give rise to a breakdown in communication and thus lead to poor patient care. Therefore, record all important steps and decisions on patient care as contemporaneously and as fully as possible, timing the entry and recording the time the event occurred. Sign, print name and indicate grade.

HUMAN RIGHTS ACT

The European Convention on Human Rights is now part of English law. Public authorities (such as NHS hospitals) must not act in a way that is incompatible with an individual's rights under the Convention including:

- Article 2 – everyone's right to life shall be protected by law
- Article 3 – inhuman or degrading treatment is prohibited
- Article 5 – all individuals have the right to liberty and security of their person save where this is sanctioned by law (e.g. lawful detention of psychiatric patients)
- Article 8 – everyone has the right to respect for their private and family life, home and correspondence
- Article 12 – men and women of marriageable age have the right to marry and found a family.

Where issues arise regarding an individual's human rights, legal advice should be sought.

ISSUES OF CLINICAL GOVERNANCE

Clinical governance is the industrial organizations' concept of total quality management mapped across medical practice. It is defined as a framework of practice where there is continuous improvement in service quality in an environment which encourages excellence in clinical care.

Well trained staff involved in regular audit and risk assessment form the cornerstones for quality care. Regular appraisal of staff to determine

---

Box 2.3 Essentials of risk management

- There is awareness of evidence based practice and its relevance.
- Procedures and advice are dispensed by medical carers with the right level of experience.
- There is continuous audit and there are continuing education programmes such as for shoulder dystocia drill and cardiotocograph interpretation.
- There is good communication between medical carers and with expectant mothers and their families. Loose talk and inadvertent comments are frequent sources for complaints.
- There is thorough and detailed address to events and outcomes surrounding every untoward incident.
- Encourage a 'no blame' culture to reinforce learning from mistakes and correct discrepancies.

competency, proper supervision and continuing education will maintain high standards of clinical capability. Constant audit of processes and procedures ensures improvement of service. Steps which will contribute to minimizing clinical risk are listed in Box 2.3.

REFERENCES

Abortion Act 1967 HMSO, London
Human Rights Act 2000 HMSO, London
Mental Health Act 1980 HMSO, London

FURTHER READING

Bolam v Friern Hospital Management Committee 1957
    1 WLR 582 Judgement of Mr Justice McNair
Department of Health 2001 Reference guide to consent for
    examination or treatment. HMSO, London
HC(90)22 A guide to consent for examination or treatment

HSG(92)32 Patient consent to examination or treatment
    model forms
Medical Defence Union 1992 Consent to Treatment. Available
    from the Medical Defence Union (MDU). Tel: 0207 486 6181
Section 124 NHS Act 1977

3

Maternal and perinatal mortality

D. Liu, C. Rodeck

Reports from Confidential Enquiries into Maternal Deaths in the UK have appeared every 3 years since 1952 and are the first example of audit by the medical profession. The Department of Health document *A First Class Service – Quality in the New NHS* (DoH 1998) states that all health workers are required to participate in these Enquiries. Information and case notes must be made available for Enquiry Assessors and reports completed within 9 months of the death. The 1994–1996 triennial audit emphasized awareness of social and public health issues. These issues include advice for seatbelt usage, identification and coordinated care for psychiatric disorders especially postnatal depression, impact of social sequestration from access to help and contribution from domestic violence.

These audits have led to substantial improvement in care and safety for childbirth. The direct maternal death rate for the 1994–1996 triennia is 6.1 per 100 000 maternities (5.0 per 100 000 maternities for 1997–1999). Mothers over 40 years, high parity, thrombo-embolism, pregnancy hypertension, amniotic fluid embolism, sepsis, haemorrhage and uterine rupture remain as salient but often avoidable causations. There is no room for complacency. Inadequate contribution and support from experienced senior obstetricians and inappropriate delegation and treatment emphasize the need for protocols, teamwork and drills to address emergencies. The continuing challenge is to achieve year on year improvement in the safety and satisfaction of childbirth, using evidence based practice.

MATERNAL MORTALITY

Maternal mortality is defined by the *International Classification of Diseases, Injuries and Causes of Death – Ninth Revision* (ICD9) (ICD9 World Health Organization Geneva 1993) as 'death of a woman while pregnant or within 42 days of termination of pregnancy from any cause related to or aggravated by the pregnancy or its management, but not from accidental or incidental causes'. This is further subdivided into the following, where maternities are defined as pregnancies which result in a live birth at any gestation or a stillbirth occurring at or after 24 completed weeks gestation (note statement for twin pregnancies, see below):

- Direct obstetric death results from obstetric complications of the pregnancy state.
- Indirect obstetric death is where existing or pregnancy precipitated medical disorders lead to or are associated with maternal mortality, for example following diabetes mellitus, cardiac diseases, vascular aneurysm, epilepsy or suicides.
- Fortuitous obstetric death is when pregnancy is incidental to the causation, for example road traffic accident, murder or unrelated malignancies.
- Late obstetric death. The *ICD10* revision introduced inclusion of direct and indirect deaths 'occurring between 42 days and 1 year after abortion, miscarriage or delivery'. The last two Confidential Enquiries included late deaths into their figures.

Causes of maternal mortality

Only direct and indirect deaths are counted for the Confidential Enquiries. The denominator is registered live or stillbirths after 24 completed weeks and not total pregnancies, since exact numbers of pregnancies are not known. International comparison is not reliable since not all countries use the same inclusion criteria. Increase in the maternal mortality figures for the 1994–1996 triennia reflected alterations in the baseline with inclusion of extra cases. Causes of death relevant to the labour ward where mortality rates have increased include pulmonary thrombo-embolism, hypertensive diseases, amniotic fluid emboli, sepsis and uterine rupture. Deaths due to anaesthesia and haemorrhage have decreased.

Substandard care continues as a contributory factor. Steps for improvement include:

- Awareness of one's limitations. Seek advice when there is uncertainty or doubt.
- Ensure delegation is appropriate for the level of competency.
- Consultants or experienced seniors must attend to assist or supervise where complications are anticipated.
- Become familiar with protocols, evidence based practice and drills for emergencies. A team approach with inclusion of relevant disciplines is essential for complex situations or emergencies.
- Where possible identify potential risk in the antenatal period.

The lowest mortality is in the second pregnancy, whilst age over 40 remains a risk factor. Ethnic groups that are socially isolated, for example new immigrants with communication difficulties, need particular attention. Psychiatric disorders are now the leading causes of maternal mortality (1997–1999).

Pulmonary thrombo-embolism and thrombosis

In the UK the pulmonary embolism rate is between 1 and 2.1 per 100 000 maternities and remains the major direct cause of maternal mortality. Most mothers survive if thrombo-embolism is treated. Failure to provide prophylaxis, to diagnose or consider possibility of diagnosis continues to place mothers at risk. The following steps should be taken to reduce risk:

- Identify family or personal history of thrombosis. Screening for thrombophilia and anti-phospholipid antibody, for example cardiolipin, Leiden factor V mutation and anti-lupus anticoagulant, may be appropriate to plan prophylaxis.

- Mothers over 35 years old weighing over 80 kg and after having 4 babies require some form of prophylaxis. Consider prophylaxis after 4 days of bed rest, when there is pre-eclampsia, dehydration and major medical illness or infection.
- Heparin prophylaxis in adequate doses in addition to stockings must be prescribed where there is a personal or family history of thrombosis, thrombophilia or where major surgery is contemplated.
- When there is suspicion or symptoms suggestive of venous thrombosis or pulmonary embolism perform Duplex ultrasound examination or ventilation-perfusion lung scan.
- Neither unfractionated nor low molecular weight heparin cross the placenta. Where risk is high prescribe unfractionated heparin 7500 units every 12 hours or equivalent. Appropriate doses must be prescribed.
- Continue prophylaxis for 5 days or until mobilized. Mothers with a history of thromboembolism need prophylaxis for 6 weeks.
- In contemporary practice all caesarean sections are covered by prophylaxis for thromboembolism.

Hypertensive disorders

The following are suggested to improve care:

- Educate medical staff and mothers concerning the significance of complications, the need for prompt attention or delivery and the benefit of a team approach in a referral centre where senior expertise is available. Proteinuria and/or hypertension can present alone before the full clinical picture.
- Clear guidelines and protocols must be in place for management of pre-eclampsia and eclampsia.
- The mortality rate ranges between 7 and 12 per million maternities. Mothers below 25 years are at particular risk. The risk also increases with age (>35 years), severe obesity and a family history of pre-eclampsia.
- An average of 6 days separates normality at antenatal review and subsequent onset of

hypertension. Ensure close liaison with GPs and community midwives since the complication can arise between antenatal visits.
- Monitor severity and progress of pre-eclampsia by full blood count, uric acid, electrolytes, liver and renal function tests. Fluid overload with pulmonary oedema and acute respiratory distress syndrome (ARDS) is a frequent cause of death. Cerebral pathology, particularly infarct and haemorrhage, is also significant.

Amniotic fluid embolism

Sudden collapse (hypotension and cardiac arrest) and cyanosis followed rapidly by death is suggestive of this complication but lung autopsy showing presence of squames and hair is needed for confirmation. Prevention is difficult but note the following:

- Strong uterine contractions, fetal distress and severe haemorrhage due to coagulopathy are other clinical features. Avoid uterine overstimulation and delay in resolving obstructed labour.
- Complication increases with age (>35 years) and high parity. Although classically associated with polyhydramnios and induction of labour with oxytocics, other obstetric complications can contribute. It is not common in a totally straightforward pregnancy but amniotic fluid embolism can present before onset of labour.

Sepsis

Puerperal sepsis has increased in the UK and is now the fourth major cause of maternal mortality. This is associated with increased virulence in streptococcal infections. To reduce risk:

- Note history of infection especially haemolytic streptococcal infections. Exclude infections in complications such as prolonged membrane rupture or presence of a cervical suture.
- Investigate promptly any pyrexia. Check full blood count. Note presence of thrombocytopenia. Obtain blood culture. Recruit help from microbiologist for severe infection. Do

not wait for culture results before instigating antibiotics.

- Prescribe prophylactic antibiotics where indicated. This is routine for caesarean section in contemporary practice.

Haemorrhage

Death due to severe haemorrhage has fallen to 3.3 per million maternities. Further improvement in management of this complication includes:

- Appropriate delegation for difficult caesarean sections such as placenta praevia, particularly when the placenta is sited anterior with a previous caesarean section scar.
- Frequent drill to familiarize with protocol for severe haemorrhage and test communication with blood banks. Recruit help from haematologists and anaesthetists. Postpartum haemorrhage (loss of 500 ml or more of blood) occurs in 1% of deliveries. Correct estimation of blood loss and being aware of clotting defect is important.
- Early resort to hysterectomy if bleeding continues despite simple procedures.
- Where risk of haemorrhage is high consider transfer of care to a tertiary unit.

Genital trauma – uterine rupture

Death rate due to uterine rupture is between 1.0 and 2.3 per million maternities. For further details see Chapter 14 and note the following when there is a uterine scar:

- An experienced obstetrician must assess suitability for vaginal delivery. Exclude risk of disproportion and pelvic anatomical deformities.
- Conduct delivery in an equipped unit with full maternal and fetal surveillance. An experienced obstetrician must supervise care of at risk pregnancies.
- Emphasize again care with oxytocic usage for induction of labour and recognition of signs and symptoms of uterine rupture.

Anaesthesia

Death rate due to anaesthesia has dropped to 0.5 per million maternities (c. 1.4 between 1997–1999). Good communication within a multidisciplinary team, availability of consultant advice and support, prompt appropriate decisions and ready access to Intensive Care Units (ICUs) will continue to reduce the contribution from anaesthesia to maternal mortality.

The labour ward is not suitable for high dependency care. The following should be noted:

- Epinephrine is the drug of choice for severe anaphylaxis.
- All medical personnel should be aware of resuscitation techniques.

PERINATAL MORTALITY

This is defined as a stillbirth from 24 weeks onwards or the death of a liveborn baby at any gestational age within 7 days of a birth (early neonatal death). Death of one twin delivered after 24 weeks is considered a stillbirth. Some countries accept the range from 20 weeks gestation to 28 days after birth, hence comparison must take definition into consideration. In England and Wales the perinatal mortality is around 9 per 1000.

Factors associated with perinatal mortality include:

- Congenital and inherited abnormalities.
- Perinatal mortality is increased after the third birth, in multiple pregnancies and where birth weight is low such as in preterm births and fetal growth restriction.
- It is increased when there are obstetric and medical complications in the mothers. Discuss mode of delivery with mothers and their partners. If vaginal delivery is appropriate close surveillance is mandatory. Process of labour can exert hypoxic stress. If there is much fetal compromise deliver by caesarean section.

More important than mortality is maternal and fetal morbidity, for which we have no detailed statistics.

REFERENCES

Department of Health 1998 A first class service – quality in the new NHS. The Department of Health, London

ICD9 1993 World Health Organization, Geneva
ICD10 1993 World Health Organization, Geneva

FURTHER READING

CESDI The Fetal and Infant Postmortem. Maternal and Child Health Consortium 2000. CESDI, London

Department of Health 1998 Why mothers die. Report on Confidential Enquiries into maternal deaths in the United Kingdom 1994–1996. The Stationery Office, London

Drife J 1997 Management of primary post partum haemorrhage. British Journal of Gynaecology 104: 275–277

Duley L 1998 Magnesium sulphate in eclampsia. Eclampsia Trial Collaborative group. Lancet 352: 67–68

Holme S E 1996 Invasive group A streptococcal infections. New England Journal of Medicine 335: 590–591

Polkinghorne J 1989 Review of the guidance on the research use of fetuses and fetal material. HMSO, London

RCOG 2001 Why mothers die 1997–1999. The Fifth Report of the Confidential Enquiries into Maternal Deaths in the United Kingdom. RCOG Press, London

The Royal College of Obstetricians and Gynaecologists 1995 Report of a working party on prophylaxis against thrombo-embolism in gynaecology and obstetrics. RCOG, London

The Scottish Office Department of Health 1998 Acute services review report. SODH TSO, The Stationery Office, Edinburgh

The Welsh Office 1998 Quality care and clinical excellence. The Welsh Office, Cardiff

4

The delivery room

A. Sullivan

Childbirth is an important and life-changing event. Creating a safe and welcoming environment for this is therefore vital. Around 98% of births in the UK take place in hospital (Chamberlain et al 1997). However, *Changing Childbirth* (DoH 1993) placed emphasis on community based care and increased partnership with mothers when making clinical decisions. One such decision is the choice concerning the place for birth. Recent policy initiatives also emphasize the need to extend choice and increase responsiveness to mothers' needs, within available resources (Honor 1997). Crucially, the effectiveness and desirability of many interventions has been questioned (RCOG and RCM 1999). The environment for birth should take account of these developments, whilst remaining mindful of the safety of all concerned.

HOSPITAL DELIVERY ROOMS

Décor

Hospital delivery rooms should be decorated to simulate some of the conditions available at home (e.g. wallpaper, borders, curtains). This may make the physical environment less clinical and threatening. The furniture should be comfortable, whilst allowing the mother to adopt a variety of positions for labour and delivery. Beanbags and floor mats may provide extra comfort. A homely atmosphere is particularly important for bereaved parents. A separate room should be provided for such circumstances.

Contents

It is important to match facilities with workload. The furniture should be comfortable for the mother, whilst allowing her to adopt a variety of positions. The bed should adapt for normal and operative deliveries. *Towards Safer Childbirth* (RCOG and RCM 1999) specifies the requirements for equipment in case of emergency. Equipment must be maintained regularly. Items are listed in Box 4.1.

There should also be prompt access to supporting facilities. These include a high-dependency unit/ICU/resuscitation facilities, depending on workload and case mix. The delivery suite should also be situated near an operating theatre. One is generally considered sufficient for up to 4000 deliveries per annum. However, units with deliveries exceeding this number should also have additional operating space. There should be prompt access to fetal blood, gas and pH analysers. Finally, an ultrasound scanner should be available.

Figure 4.1 shows a typical delivery room.

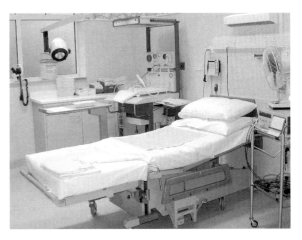

Figure 4.1 Example of a delivery room.

Box 4.1 Equipment for delivery rooms

Maternal resuscitation
- Oxygen and suction
- Bed available for prompt resuscitation

Fetal wellbeing
- 2–4 CTG machines/1000 deliveries (one capable of monitoring twins)
- Equipment for intermittent fetal auscultation (Pinards/Doppler/Sonicaid)

Neonatal resuscitation (usually contained within a Resuscitaire)
- Resuscitation surface, overhead radiant heat source, stop clock, suction device and catheters, stethoscope
- Oxygen/air supply with variable regulated flow rate and adjustable pressure-relief valve, Y-piece or 500 ml self-inflating resuscitation bag, valve and face masks
- 2 laryngoscopes with straight blades (appropriate sizes)
- Tracheal tubes (2.5, 3.0 and 4.0 mm)
- Syringes, scissors, umbilical vessel catheterization pack, nasogastric tubes sizes 5 and 8, intravenous cannulae
- Checklist, resuscitation flow chart/algorithm

The use of water immersion for labour and delivery

Water immersion is now used in a wide range of hospital and community settings. Research findings concerning its safety and efficacy remain inconclusive and even conflicting (Hartley 1998). However, the RCM Position Statement (RCM 1995) states that, on balance, water birth appears safe and should be offered to childbearing women. Many hospitals have a purpose-built room for water birth.

The potential benefits of water birth include:

- relaxant effects and reduced need for pharmacological analgesia (Burns and Greenish 1993)
- shorter labour with increased perineal elasticity (Burns and Greenish 1993) and
- reduced perineal trauma (Gordon 1996).

Potential hazards include:

- higher incidence of postpartum haemorrhage, due to increased maternal vasodilatation (Eldering & Selke 1996)
- increased maternal and fetal infection (Gordon 1996)
- water inhalation by the fetus (Johnson 1996)
- delay instigating emergency interventions (Nikodem 1997) and
- increased intrapartum asphyxia, secondary to maternal hyperthermia (Charles 1998).

Only the latter has been substantiated. Current recommendations therefore state that pool temperature is carefully monitored and is not allowed to exceed normal body temperature. Requirements for water birth safety are listed in Box 4.2.

The equipment needed for a water birth is shown in Figure 4.2.

Box 4.2   Requirements for water birth

Infection control
- Disinfection of pool and all equipment after each use
- Tap water is safe, but should not enter and exit the pool via the same aperture (any tubing should also be sterilized)

Maternal and fetal wellbeing
- No electrical sockets installed (treat as a bathroom)
- Only low-risk mothers should use the pool (according to locally agreed criteria)
- Hourly monitoring of maternal and pool temperature
- Maternal and fetal observations as for any low-risk labour
- Delivery bed and resuscitation equipment should be readily available
- Equipment to lift the mother out of the pool in emergency (e.g. reinforced net)

Issues for staff
- Adequate training should be provided, with clear guidelines for practice
- Attention to manual handling issues (back care)
- Awareness of action in emergency, including tight nuchal cord, shoulder dystocia and maternal collapse)

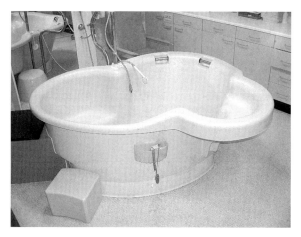

Figure 4.2   Equipment for a water birth.

HOME DELIVERY

There is no convincing evidence that hospital births are safest for mothers and babies (House of Commons Committee 1992). Some mothers may prefer to deliver at home because of the convenience of being in one's own environment, reduced interference in labour and increased freedom of choice (Chamberlain et al 1997). However, planned home delivery is only thought to be advisable for low-risk mothers and the midwife should be trained and comfortable in the home environment (Hall 1999). There should also be robust and clear guidelines concerning transfer to hospital where problems arise (RCOG and RCM 1999). The midwife should recognize when this is necessary and act accordingly. In the main, obstetric and paediatric flying squads have been replaced by paramedics. These principles are also appropriate for midwifery-managed delivery units. The equipment required for home delivery is listed in Box 4.3.

Box 4.3   Equipment for home delivery

- Access to a mobile phone or telephone within the home
- Room heater and good light, towels and gloves
- Self-inflating resuscitation bag, valve and face masks of appropriate sizes
- Suction device and catheters, resuscitation flow chart, stop watch, stethoscope
- Oxygen cylinder with regulated flow rate of up to 10 L/min and adjustable pressure-relief valve
- Syringes, needles and disposal box, checklist
- Pinards/Doppler/Sonicaid
- Sterile gloves, amnihook, lubricating jelly, equipment for suturing
- Thermometers, Entonox, measuring jug, sphygmomanometer, oxytocic drugs
- Urinary catheter, urine testing equipment, torch, tourniquet, cord clamp
- Scales, birth notification forms

PSYCHOLOGICAL REQUIREMENTS FOR THE PLACE OF BIRTH

Although the physical environment is important for the safety and wellbeing of those involved with a birth, the atmosphere created by staff is also vital. Carers should be pleasant and relaxed, whilst remaining as unobtrusive as possible. Mothers and their chosen companions will then be allowed to share the experience with maximum dignity. Teaching hospitals require students to gain experience, but the wishes of the mother should be considered. At times, gender issues may arise and mothers and their partners may request female attendants. Where possible, the wishes of parents should be respected (Nicum & Karoo 1998). Finally, it is essential to develop good working relationships between members of the multidisciplinary team involved in the mother's care. A spirit of collaboration and clear lines of communication can significantly enhance mothers' perceptions of their birth environment in a positive light.

REFERENCES

Burns E, Greenish K 1993 Pooling information. Nursing Times 89(8): 47–49

Chamberlain G, Wraight A, Crowley P 1997 Home births. The report of the 1994 Confidential Enquiry by National Birthday Trust Fund. Parthenon, USA

Charles C 1998 Fetal hyperthermia risk from warm water immersion. British Journal of Midwifery 6(3): 152–156

Department of Health 1993 Changing childbirth. Report of the Expert Maternity Group. HMSO, London

Eldering G, Selke K 1996 Water birth – a possible mode of delivery. In: Beech B (ed) Waterbirth unplugged. Books For Midwives Press, Cheshire, p 19–33

Gordon Y 1996 Water birth – the safety issues. In: Beech B (ed) Waterbirth unplugged. Books For Midwives Press, Cheshire, p 135–142

Hall J 1999 Home birth: the midwife effect. British Journal of Midwifery 7(4): 225–227

Hartley J 1998 The use of water during labour and birth. RCM Midwives Journal 1(12): 366–369

Honor P 1997 Review of the maternity services 1996/7. District Audit, Southampton

House of Commons Health Committee 1992 Maternity Services Second Report (Winterton Report). HMSO, London

Johnson P 1996 Birth under water – to breathe or not to breathe. British Journal of Obstetrics and Gynaecology 103(3): 202–208

Nicum R, Karoo R 1998 Expectations and opinions of pregnant women about medical students being involved in care at the time of delivery. Medical Education (32)3: 320–324

Nikodem V 1997 Immersion in water during pregnancy, labour and birth. In: Neilson J, Crowther C, Hodnett E, Hofmeyr G (eds) Pregnancy and childbirth module of the Cochrane database of systematic reviews. The Cochrane Collaboration, Issue 4

Royal College of Midwives 1995 The use of water during birth: position statement. RCM, London

Royal College of Obstetricians and Gynaecologists and Royal College of Midwives 1999 Towards safer childbirth. Minimum standards for the organisation of labour wards. Report of the RCOG/RCM working parties. RCOG/RCM, London

5

Admission to the labour ward

D. Liu

ADMISSION FOR LABOUR

The modern labour ward subserves many functions. It is a place where mothers can self admit or are referred for assessment and reviewed by a well equipped obstetric team when there are anxieties or complications associated with their pregnancies, for example suspected preterm labour, membrane rupture or abdominal pain.

Requirements for care are:

- Take detailed history. Review obstetric and gynaecological history.
- If appropriate, consult colleagues in other medical disciplines.
- Perform thorough examination of mother and fetus. This can include cardiotocograph record and ultrasound scan for reassurance.
- Reassure and allow home if there is no evidence of complication. Where necessary arrange follow-up appointments to ensure continuity of care.
- Admit to the antenatal ward for observation or treatment if there are medical or obstetric reasons. There is a place for admission to promote a caring attitude when mothers' anxieties are not resolved.

The labour ward is also a place for emergency care of expectant mothers. Reasons for admission include medical emergencies, for example status asthmaticus or myocardial infarction, and obstetric complications, for example antepartum haemorrhage or eclampsia. When an emergency situation arises:

- Address emergency. Stabilize the mother's condition.
- Recruit support from appropriate colleagues such as anaesthetists, haematologists, physicians or surgeons. Where possible consult colleagues with particular interest in obstetrics.
- Address obstetric emergencies (Ch. 6).
- Document clearly in detail all steps undertaken. This retrospective record is made as soon as possible, when memories of events are still fresh in mind.
- Keep partners and accompanying persons fully informed.
- Any emergency is a frightening situation. Efficient professionalism contributes much to a calm atmosphere and reduces anxiety.

Organizational requirements

The various functions of the labour ward demand a sound organization structure to provide effective care. Requirements include:

- A lead clinician with particular interest in the labour ward.
- A labour ward forum which meets on a regular basis (for example weekly) to encompass audit, teaching, health and safety and risk management issues.
- Close liaison with neonatologists.
- Frequent drills and regular updating to anticipate emergencies, for example shoulder dystocia or haemorrhage, to ensure provision of evidence based care. Ability to interpret cardiotocograph traces is essential.
- Levels of staffing must be adequate. A robust process for induction of new staff of all levels, regular appraisal and continued education programmes must be in place.
- A senior obstetrician supervises and must be readily available to advise and support. The ideal is a move towards consultant based care for complicated pregnancies whilst midwives will attend to normal deliveries.

Requirements for quality care

Cultural changes prompted by better information, national (e.g. Expert Maternity Group 1993) and international (e.g. NHMRC 1996) directives and surveys indicate that mothers and their partners expect quality and satisfaction in addition to safe delivery. There is evidence to show the following contribute to perceived quality and satisfaction:

- Rapport and satisfaction during antenatal care.
- A welcoming attitude at the time of admission.
- There is good communication. Mothers and partners are kept well informed at all stages and encouraged to participate in care decisions.
- Provide reassurance, encouragement and good pain relief. These steps are essential if active labour unexpectedly extends beyond 12 hours.
- Limit the number of persons in the delivery room at any one time. Respect the need for privacy.
- Ensure continuity of care expectations even if the carer changes. Not all personal midwives can stay for the whole duration of labour.
- Be as helpful as possible.
- Take note of the choice of language used for communication.
- Limit use of episiotomies.

Labour is the most common reason for admission.

- Obtain detailed history to determine diagnosis for onset of labour, the state of the fetal membranes and the presence of mucoid show.
- Consider the differential diagnosis for intermittent abdominal pain, vaginal bleeding and leakage of fluid from the vagina (e.g. urinary incontinence or infection).
- Review the antenatal history. Knowledge of antenatal history is particularly important when mothers ring in for advice. Document main points of conversation.
- Reassure once the correct diagnosis of labour has been established.

ASSESSMENT FOLLOWING ADMISSION

Presentation

This describes the fetal part presented or nearest to the cervix, e.g. cephalic presentation.

Lie

This defines the relationship between the longitudinal axis of the fetus and that of the mother (Fig. 5.1).

Engagement

This occurs when the biparietal (vertex) or biischial (breech) diameters descend below the pelvic brim. Descent of the fetal head into the pelvis is usually described as if the head is divided into five segments. The head would be engaged if less than three-fifths were palpable above the pelvic brim (Fig. 5.2).

Examination of abdomen and pelvis

- Place mother on her back, with her head on a single pillow, her hands by her sides and both knees slightly bent. The bladder should be empty. Use semirecumbent position if supine hypotension troubles.

- Note the general health and clinical condition, e.g. generalized oedema. Record temperature, pulse, blood pressure and examine urine for presence of protein, ketones, sugar and blood.
- Observe and note the shape and contour of the abdomen.
- Note the frequency, duration and intensity of uterine contractions.
- Stand on the mother's right side, maintain rapport by conversation and watch her facial expression as a guide to inadvertent cause of discomfort during palpation.
- Warm hands and palpate the abdomen gently to estimate the gestational age by fundal height, approximate fetal size, lie, presentation, amount of liquor and engagement of the presenting part.

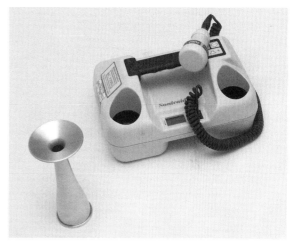

Figure 5.3 Pinard stethoscope and Doppler fetal heart rate detector.

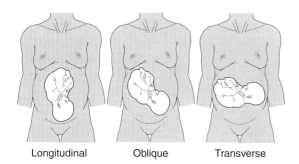

Longitudinal   Oblique   Transverse

Figure 5.1   Longitudinal, oblique and transverse lie.

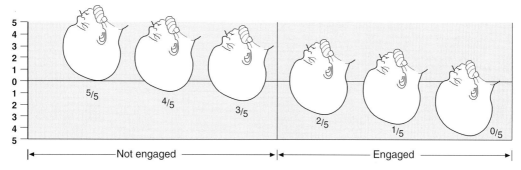

Figure 5.2   Engagement described in fifths. Left non-engaged, right engaged.

- Place hand on the fundus or measure to estimate fundal height. Percuss if there is difficulty locating upper limit of uterus. Fundal height can be only a rough guide to gestational age (Fig. 5.4).

  Many physical features, such as the mother's stature, affect estimation of gestation by fundal height. Take into account the weight of the mother and her partner, when they were born and the size of the previous babies. A reduction in fundal height in primigravidae near term is due to engagement of the presenting part.

- Auscultate with Pinard stethoscope or Doppler heart detector (Fig. 5.3). Fetal heart sound is loudest over the anterior fetal shoulder (Fig. 5.5). Listen through a contraction to exclude late fetal heart rate deceleration.

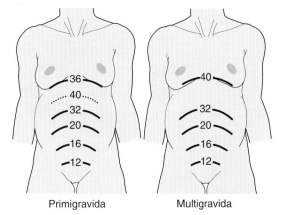

Primigravida   Multigravida

Figure 5.4   Fundal height in primigravida and multigravida.

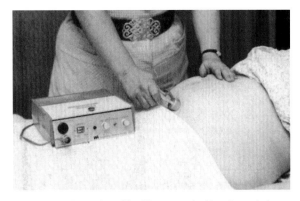

Figure 5.5   Detection of fetal heart rate by Doppler technique.

- Perform speculum examination (Box 5.1) if indicated.
- If the membranes are ruptured, note the colour of the amniotic fluid and whether meconium or blood staining is present. Take samples for culture if the membranes have been ruptured for more than 6 hours.
- Note application of the presenting part of the fetus to the cervix. Exclude cord prolapse.

Cervical examination

- The cervix dilates in concentric circles from a diameter of less than 1 cm to full dilatation of 10 cm. Estimate cervical dilatation (Fig. 5.8).
- The cervix is essentially a thick cylinder of collagen. Before dilatation can occur a process of thinning and shortening, or effacement, must take place. During pregnancy and early labour physiological changes are directed towards softening of the cervix (Fig. 5.9).

  Effacement reflects the existence of uterine activity and indicates the ease and readiness of the cervix to dilate. Once the effaced cervix can no longer resist uterine contractions, dilatation begins.

- Before removal of the speculum check for normality of the cervix, for the presence of vaginal infection and for evidence of varicosities. When indicated take cervical swabs. Learn to recognize presence of active herpes infection.

Vaginal examination

- Use full aseptic precautions.
- Warn mother of what to expect.
- Insert index and, if that is tolerated, middle finger through introitus.
- Palpate around the fornices and sense the proximity of the presenting part of the fetus to the examining finger. A spongy feel interposed between the finger and the presenting part warns of the possibility of undiagnosed placenta praevia.
- Confirm observed cervical dilatation. The number of fingers accommodated by the cervix can be used as a measure, e.g. four

---

Box 5.1   Speculum examination

Pass speculum (Fig. 5.6) with full aseptic precautions to examine the cervix.

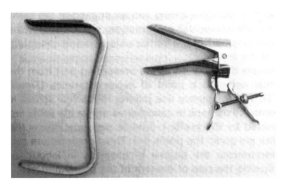

Figure 5.6   Speculums in common use: Sim's (left), Cusco's (right).

Step 1
Explain the need for examination, cleanse the vulval area, indicate your intention before insertion of the instrument.

Cusco's speculum: Step 2
Insert the speculum with the blades closed and in line with opening of the introitus for 3–4 cm, rotate so the handle is towards the sacrum, warn mother of the sensation of pressure as the speculum is opened.

Step 3
Advance speculum to locate cervix.

Sim's speculum: Step 2
Insert the speculum 3–4 cm maintaining direction towards the sacrum. Warn the mother of sensation of pressure as speculum is gently pulled backwards to view cervix (Fig. 5.7).

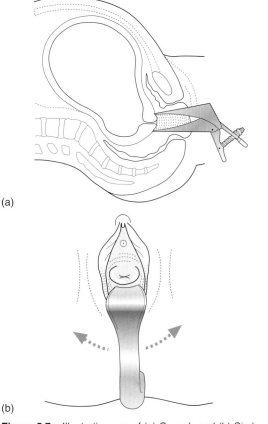

(a)

(b)

Figure 5.7   Illustrating use of (a) Cusco's and (b) Sim's speculum.

Step 3
Consider the position of the fourchette to be 6 o'clock. Move the speculum through an arc between 5 and 7 o'clock to obtain a better view. Displace the anterior vaginal wall with sponge forceps if necessary.

---

fingers indicates full dilatation; one fingerbreadth is approximately 1.5 cm.
- Feel for fetal membranes. If the membranes are ruptured exclude cord prolapse. If the membranes are intact palpate to exclude pulsations due to cord presentation or vasa praevia. When active labour is present and the cervix is 4 cm or more dilated the membranes can be ruptured to facilitate labour. A scalp 'clip' for electronic fetal heart rate monitoring can be applied at the same time. Determine the presentation, application of the presenting part of the fetus and length and consistency of the cervix.
- Estimate the distance of the presenting part from the ischial spine as a point of pelvic reference (Fig. 5.10). The imaginary line joining the ischial spines is station 0. Positions

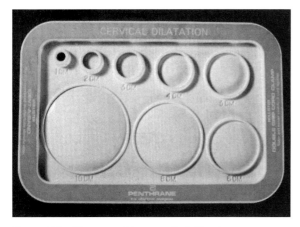

Figure 5.8   Plate as guide to cervical dilatation.

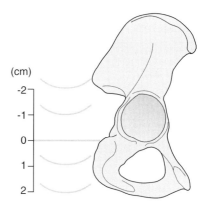

Figure 5.10   Pelvic landmarks as rough guides to level of presenting parts.

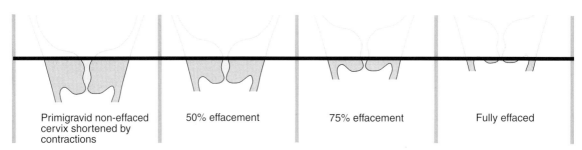

| Primigravid non-effaced cervix shortened by contractions | 50% effacement | 75% effacement | Fully effaced |

Figure 5.9   Cross-section of cervix to illustrate the degree of effacement.

in centimetres above the spine are denoted by the prefix – while positions below the spine are given the prefix +. This nomenclature can communicate the amount of progress in labour by indicating the rate of descent of the presenting part.

Information acquired at this stage of examination can be expressed collectively as a score, which was first introduced by Bishop (1964). Table 5.1 shows a modified version of this. A score of more than 5 reflects ease of cervical dilatation.

- In cephalic presentation, locate and note direction of the sagittal suture. Identify the anterior and posterior fontanelle (Fig. 5.11). The posterior fontanelle dimples in the shape of a 'V' where the three sutures meet, whilst the anterior fontanelle is larger, the surrounding bones feel less firm, and can be followed out to four sutures. A readily palpable anterior

Table 5.1   Modified Bishop cervical score

Cervix	Score			
	0	1	2	3
Dilatation (cm)	Closed	1–2	3–4	>5
Length (cm)	3	2	1	0
Consistency	Firm	Medium	Soft	
Position	Posterior	Middle	Anterior	
Station of head (cm)	–3	–2	–1–0	+1–+2

fontanelle indicates poor head flexion. Identification of sutures is made more difficult by oedema of the fetal scalp or caput succedaneum.

Pelvic examination

Develop a routine for examination which is thorough, gentle and quick. During examination bear in mind the following:

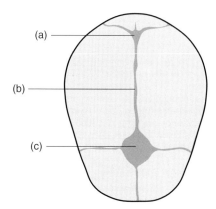

Figure 5.11   (a) Posterior fontanelle, (b) sagittal suture, (c) anterior fontanelle.

Table 5.2   Average diameters of the normal pelvis (cm)

	Anteroposterior	Transverse	Oblique
Brim	12	12	12
Cavity	12	12	12
Outlet	12	11.5	12

into consideration ethnic differences and gestation. Suspicion should be aroused when:

- congenital skeletal defect is present
- the mother is of short stature
- there is a history of pelvic trauma (e.g. road traffic accident)
- there is evidence of dietary or medical diseases affecting bone formation (e.g. tuberculosis or osteomyelitis).

Routine for pelvic examination

A useful routine for pelvic assessment is given below:

- Tell mother of your intent and warn her that some pressure may be felt.
- Introduce fingers through the introitus and press against the subpubic arch (Fig. 5.15). If the arch accommodates two fingers comfortably (more than 90°) then the pelvis is likely to be gynaecoid or platypelloid.
- Locate the ischial spines, note their prominence and depth from symphysis to anterior half of the pelvis (Fig. 5.16).
- Keeping the third finger in contact with the ischial spine, move the index finger along the sacrospinous ligament and gauge the width of the sacrosiatic notch. The notch, which indicates the depth of the posterior half of the pelvis, is wide if the sacrum is 3 cm or more from the ischial spine.

- The four basic pelvic types: gynaecoid, android, ellipsoid and platypelloid. With experience combinations of these basic types can be identified.

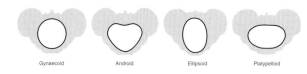

- The various pelvic planes (Box 5.2). The plane of least pelvic diameter describes the narrowest part of the pelvis.
- The two narrowest diameters are the interischial (10.5 cm) and the transverse diameter of the outlet (11.5 cm).
- Any diameter which is less than 9.5 cm is not adequate for a normal full term fetus. Absolute disproportion is present.
- Knowledge of the length of the examiner's fingers and width of the knuckles is useful.
- There are ethnic differences. All pelvic diameters in mothers of smaller stature may be reduced by 0.5–1 cm.

The average diameters of the normal pelvis are given in Table 5.2.

Contracted pelvis

This is suspected when any of the above diameters is reduced by more than 1 cm. Take

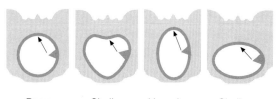

Deep   Shallow   Very deep   Shallow

Box 5.2 Pelvic planes

Diameters of pelvic planes are shown in Figure 5.12. Anteroposterior diameters of the pelvis are shown in Figure 5.13.

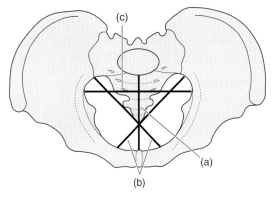

Figure 5.12 Pelvic diameters: (a) anteroposterior, (b) oblique, (c) transverse. In each case the widest diameter is chosen.

(a) True conjugate = promontory to innermost posterior surface of symphysis (measured in erect lateral pelvimetry).
(b) Diagonal conjugate = promontory to lower border of symphysis pubis (measured clinically).
(c) Anteroposterior diameter of outlet = lower border of symphysis pubis to end of sacrum (measured clinically and radiologically).

Pelvic planes are shown in Figure 5.14.

(a) Brim or inlet – upper border of symphysis pubis, iliopectineal line, sacrum.
(b) Midcavity or greatest pelvic diameter – midpoint of posterior symphysis, upper aspect of sacrosiatic notch, junction of second and third sacral vertebrae. This is above plane of least diameter.
(c) Least pelvic diameter – mid-symphysis pubis, ischial spines, sacrospinous ligament and tip of sacrum. This is the narrowest part of the pelvis.
(d) Outlet – this plane is made up of two segments angled at the intertuberous diameter. Lower border of the symphysis, pubic arch, ischial tuberosity, sacrotuberous ligament and tip of coccyx.

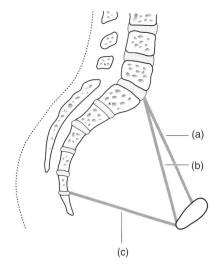

Figure 5.13 Anteroposterior diameters of the pelvis: (a) true conjugate, (b) diagonal conjugate, (c) anteroposterior diameter of outlet.

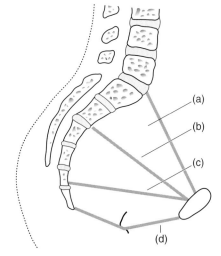

Figure 5.14 Pelvic planes: (a) brim (inlet), (b) midcavity (greatest pelvic diameter), (c) least pelvic diameter and (d) outlet.

- Repeat this procedure on the opposite side of the pelvis. Make a mental note of the distance between the spines.
- Determine whether the promontory is palpable.

It is not necessary to touch the promontory if the length of the examining finger is known. An engaged presenting part prevents examination but signifies an adequate inlet (Fig. 5.17).

- Sweep the fingers along the sacral curve. Note any reduction in curvature or protrusion of the sacrum into the pelvic cavity.
- Test the mobility of the coccyx.
- Withdraw the fingers. Clench them and measure intertuberous diameter with the knuckle of the hand. Take into account the shape of the

pubis. Note the distance from the tuberosity to the tip of the sacrum. This distance indicates the room available in outlet if the subpubic arch is narrowed (Fig. 5.18).

The above procedure need take no more than one minute and provides a comprehensive picture of pelvic diameters. What is not known is the mobility of the pelvis at lumbosacral and symphysial joints.

Table 5.3 summarizes the four basic pelvic configurations.

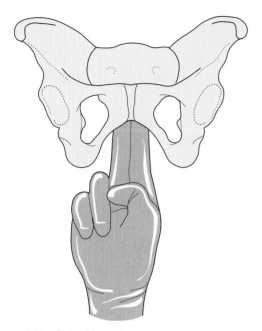

Figure 5.15　Subpubic angle.

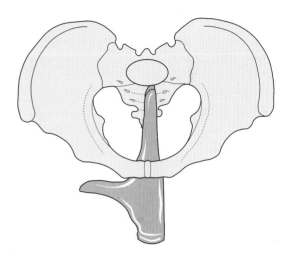

Figure 5.17　Diagonal conjugate.

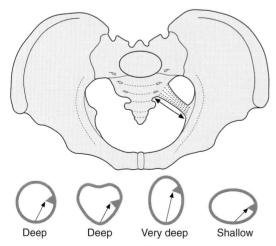

Deep　Deep　Very deep　Shallow

Figure 5.16　Ischial spine and length of sacrospinous ligament.

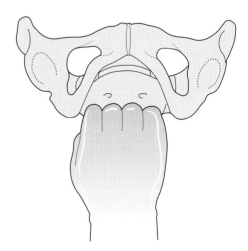

Figure 5.18　Intertuberous diameter.

Table 5.3 Summary of four basic pelvic configurations

Type	Gynaecoid	Android	Ellipsoid	Platypelloid
Incidence	50%	20%	25%	5%
Geometrical shape	◯	▽	⬭	⬭
Subpubic angle	>90°	<90°	<90°	>90°
Ischial spines	Not prominent	Prominent	Usually not prominent	Can be prominent
Sacrosiatic notch	Wide	Narrow	Wide	Wide
Interspinous diameter	Wide	Narrow	Narrow	Wide
Pelvic walls	Parallel	Convergent	Parallel	Divergent
Intertuberous diameter	Wide	Reduced	Reduced	Wide

Erect lateral pelvimetry (ELP)

When disproportion is suspected an upright lateral radiographic view (Fig. 5.19) or magnetic resonance image (MRI) (Fig. 5.20) of the pelvis provides additional information.

For interpretation of ELP or MRI of the pelvis the following should be carried out:

- Check that the femoral trochanters are aligned.
- Check the presentation and position of the fetus. Density of the fetal bones gives an indication of their maturity.
- Count the number of sacral vertebrae. Note the degree of curvature of the sacrum and the length of the coccyx. Sacralization of the fifth lumbar vertebra (inclusion of the fifth lumbar vertebra into the sacrum) increases the depth of the pelvis and impedes engagement.

- Measure the true conjugate and the antero-posterior diameter of outlet. Pelvic convergence is readily identified.
- Inclination of the pelvis is normally 55° (range 40–60°). The greater the angle of inclination the more difficult it is for engagement to take place, signifying the possibility of a longer labour (Fig. 5.21). The angle of inclination is the angle made by the line joining the promontory, the upper border of the symphysis and the horizontal plane.
- ELP assesses adequacy of the pelvis in one plane only. The width of the pelvis must be determined before adequacy is pronounced. An MRI provides three-dimensional measurements.

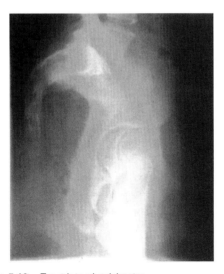

Figure 5.19 Erect lateral pelvimetry.

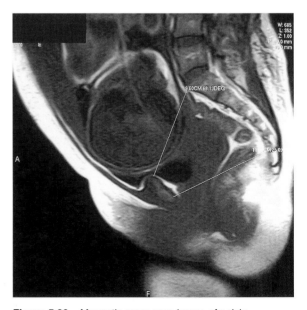

Figure 5.20 Magnetic resonance image of pelvis.

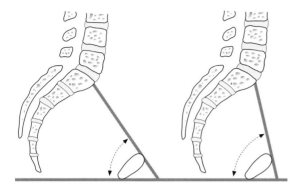

Figure 5.21   Increased inclination presents less favourable angle for entry to pelvis.

SUBSEQUENT MANAGEMENT

When complications are excluded and further labour is safe, note the following:

- If labour is in its early stages and the cervix is less than 3 cm dilated, the bowels can be emptied with suppositories. Mothers usually feel more comfortable after this procedure and there is less risk of faecal contamination. If there is no contraindication the mother can remain ambulant.
- The perineum is seldom shaved nowadays.
- Mothers in active labour frequently prefer to lie in bed.
- Safety must dictate choice for alternative mode of delivery, e.g. into water.

REFERENCES

Bishop E H 1964 Pelvic scoring for elective induction. Obstetrics and Gynecology 24: 266

Expert Maternity Group 1993 Changing childbirth: The report of the expert maternity group (Cumberlege Report). HMSO, London

National Health and Medical Research Council 1996 Report on options for effective care in childbirth. NHMRC, Canberra

FURTHER READING

Brown S, Lumley J 1998 Changing childbirth: lessons from an Australian survey of 1336 women. British Journal of Obstetrics and Gynaecology 105: 143–155

Carr-Hill R 1992 The measurement of patient satisfaction. Journal of Public Health Medicine 14: 236–249

Department of Health 1998 Why mothers die. Report on confidential enquiries into maternal deaths in the United Kingdom 1994–1996. The Stationery Office, London

House of Commons Select Committee on Health 1992 Second report on maternity services (Winterton Report). HMSO, London

Royal College of Obstetricians and Gynaecologists and Royal College of Midwives 1999 Towards safer childbirth, minimum standards for the organisation of labour wards. RCOG/RCM, RCOG Press, London

6

Admission emergencies

D. Liu, K. Ismail, M. Kilby

When emergencies occur a well rehearsed approach facilitates efficient teamwork and ensures that all correct steps are taken. The availability of clear, updated protocols is crucial for immediate management by staff on the labour ward.

Training protocols or drills for staff (doctors, midwives, anaesthetists, paediatricians and theatre assistants) are encouraged for improving performance and outcome in emergencies.

MANAGEMENT OF IMMINENT DELIVERY WITH OR WITHOUT FETAL COMPROMISE

The following procedures should be adopted if delivery is imminent:

- Determine at once whether vaginal delivery is **feasible** and **safe.**
- **Reassurance.** These mothers are often agitated and distressed on admission to hospital. Reassurance and supportive care are necessary. Discourage pushing until vaginal examination is performed.
- Transfer mother to the delivery room if vaginal delivery is safe. If fetal distress is present, expedite delivery and anticipate the need for neonatal resuscitation.
- If there is indication for or need for recurrent caesarean section proceed to immediate delivery by caesarean section. For uncomplicated cephalic presentation a period of close observation is acceptable, but anticipate assisted delivery if there is delay or onset of compromise.

SPECIFIC PROBLEMS
Cord presentation or prolapse

Always confirm **gestational age** before planning any further management.

Cord presentation

This occurs when the cord is in front of the presenting part of the fetus behind intact membranes. Whenever the membranes are not ruptured, palpate through them with the tip of the fingers to exclude the presence of pulsation due to cord presentation or vasa praevia (Fig. 6.1a). The diagnosis can also be made using ultrasound and colour flow Doppler and is useful in circumstances such as an unstable breech presentation.

Management

- Cord presentation during labour and before full cervical dilatation necessitates delivery by caesarean section.
- If the cervix is fully dilated, the presenting part is below the ischial spines and the pelvis is adequate, rupture the membranes, displace the cord and deliver by forceps or ventouse.

Cord prolapse

Following membrane rupture the cord may prolapse through the cervix, may remain in the vagina or may be expelled through the introitus (Fig. 6.1b).

Cord prolapse occurs in approximately 0.2% of all births.

Risk factors for cord prolapse

- Low birthweight (<2.5 kg)
- Premature birth
- Malpresentations
- Second twin
- High presenting part.

Points to remember in management

- Anticipate in the presence of risk factors.
- Inform the mother of the situation and the need for urgency.

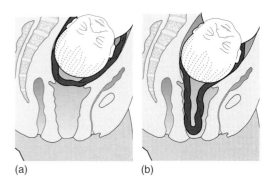

(a)   (b)

Figure 6.1 (a) Cord presentation and (b) cord prolapse.

- Check the presence of pulsation, replace the cord in the warmth of the vagina and determine dilatation of the cervix.
- Maternal O_2, intravenous (IV) access and group and save if appropriate.
- Deliver by forceps or ventouse if cervix is fully dilated and vaginal delivery is considered to be safe.
- If the cervix is not fully dilated, displace the presenting part of the fetus away from the cervix with examining digits to prevent cord compression. This manoeuvre is made easier if the mother is placed in the Trendelenburg or knee–chest position. Some authors advocate a temporary measure by inserting a number 16 Foley catheter to fill the bladder with 500 ml of saline using a standard infusion set. Bladder filling raises the presenting part of the fetus away from the cord.
- Avoid handling the cord because this will cause spasm of the vessels and fetal bradycardia.
- Request assistance and organize a theatre for caesarean section if vaginal delivery is not considered safe.

Major obstetric haemorrhage

- Haemorrhage remains one of the leading causes of maternal mortality worldwide. It is the leading cause of maternal mortality in developing countries.
- Defined as the loss of more than 500 ml blood either ante partum or post partum.
- Accurate measurement of blood loss is difficult hence a definition based on volume alone

has shortcomings. Tachycardia, hypotension, peripheral vasoconstriction and decreased urine output are important signs.

- Underestimation of blood loss may delay steps to prepare for or prevent further bleeding.

Management

- Clear guidelines must be available for haemorrhage. These will include details for contact of senior obstetric staff, anaesthetists and haematologist.
- Adequate tissue perfusion is essential to preserve organ function.
- Hypotension mediated endothelial damage may trigger disseminated intravascular coagulation (DIC).
- Basic resuscitation procedures include
  — minimize effects of aortocaval compression (left lateral tilt or wedging 5–15°
  — administer a high concentration of O_2 to the mother regardless of her oxygen saturation
  — assess **A**irway and **B**reathing effort. Intubation may be indicated if the mother has depressed conscious level due to hypotension (near arrest scenario)
  — establish two 14 G intravenous lines and take 20 ml blood for diagnostic test (full blood count, urea and electrolytes, coagulation screen and cross matching)
  — maintain the **C**irculation by normal/saline or Hartmann's solutions and colloid until blood is available.
- Monitor pulse, blood pressure (direct or indirect), respiratory rate, oxygen saturation, urine output and fluid balance.
- Central venous pressure (CVP) monitoring is recommended. Use anticubital fossa and long line as safer when coagulopathy threatens. Fluid warmers and high pressure infusers are helpful in these situations. If CVP is more than 5 mmHg maintenance of fluid volume is sufficient.
- Identify and treat the cause of bleeding.

Box 6.1 gives details of blood component therapy.

> **Box 6.1** Blood component therapy
>
> - O negative blood should be available in the delivery suite. This carries a small risk of sensitization to 'c' antigen.
> - Full infection screen is necessary for fresh whole blood.
> - After 48 hours storage, platelet numbers and function of important clotting factors (V and VIII) are reduced.
> - Full cross match of blood may take up to an hour.
> - Fresh frozen plasma (FFP) is separated from whole blood within 6 hours of donation and stored for up to one year at −20°C to −30°C. FFP provides all necessary clotting factors. Give 1 unit after 8 units of rapidly transfused blood. Use coagulation screen as guide.
> - Cryoprecipitat contains more fibrinogen than FFP but lacks antithrombin III (coagulation inhibitor), which is depleted in obstetric related coagulopathies. Cryoprecipitat is useful for hypofibrinogenaemia.
> - Platelet packs have a limited shelf life of 5 days and should be given through a platelet filter. Rarely indicated above a platelet count of 50×10^9/l.
> - In the presence of maternal antibodies, blood should be cross matched before onset of labour or caesarean section.

Antepartum haemorrhage

This is vaginal bleeding after a gestational age of 24 weeks. Bleeding is due to:

- Placental abruption or separation of the placenta which is normally situated in the upper uterine segment.
- Placenta praevia or separation of the abnormally situated placenta which lies in or encroaches onto the lower uterine segment.
- Non-placental causes secondary to trauma, infection or neoplasms.
- Vasa praevia. Bleeding is associated with rupture of blood vessels in the fetal membranes. Fetal blood is lost. Abnormal cord insertion or succenturate placenta is commonly found. The Apt test can be used if bleeding of fetal origin is suspected. The basis of this test is that fetal haemoglobin is alkaline stable, whereas adult haemoglobin is not.

Important points to remember about vaginal bleeding in pregnancy

- A show is diagnosed only when blood-stained mucus is noted, usually in association with contractions. Presence of pure blood is not a show.

- A high presenting part or malpresentation on abdominal examination may be due to placenta praevia (irrespective of an early pregnancy ultrasound scan).
- A tense contracted tender uterus is one of the signs of placental abruption.
- Vaginal examination is contraindicated until placenta praevia is excluded.
- The fetus can contribute to the bleeding hence the real risk of exsanguination.
- Bleeding is often more extensive than that observed.
- Increased uterine activity can produce or follow placental separation.
- Anti-D for rhesus negative mothers – use Kleihauer test.
- Anticipate postpartum haemorrhage.
- Ultrasound scan may detect retroplacental collection of blood.
- Placental damage and thromboplastin release can cause coagulation defect.

General guidelines for management

- Apply general rule for resuscitation (**A**irway, **B**reathing and **C**irculation + O$_2$)
- Ensure IV access (at least 16 G, preferably 14 G).
- Perform full blood count, group and cross match blood (number of units required depends on amount of bleeding).
- Exclude placenta praevia by ultrasound scan. Check fetal viability.
- Perform speculum examination (if no placenta praevia) to exclude local causes for bleeding.
- Take vaginal swab to screen for infection.
- Commence cardiotocography to assess fetal wellbeing. Further placental separation can occur. Do not stop monitoring too early.

- Note presence or absence of uterine activity.
- Clot lysis suggests activation of fibrinolytic system.

Modify guidelines for various degree of antepartum haemorrhage.

Placental separation (abruption)

Presentation depends on the amount of bleeding (Table 6.1).

Diagnosis

- A careful history should be taken to define obstetric complications, the site of pain and if coitus had taken place.
- Exclude differential diagnosis.
- If pain is not localized to the placental site concealed haemorrhage is less likely.
- Note the presence of uterine activity.
- Ultrasound examination is helpful for assessing fetal wellbeing, placental localization and identifying retroplacental haematoma.
- A negative scan does not exclude the diagnosis of abruption.
- Major placental separation produces the classical picture of shock, a rock hard uterus, coagulation defects and fetal death (in 50% of cases).
- Uterine tenderness and rigidity may be absent if the placenta is posterior.
- Haematuria may be present.
- There is an association with pre-eclampsia (2%).

Management

This is governed by the amount of bleeding, whether bleeding continues, the state of both the mother and fetus, the gestational age of the pregnancy and previous obstetric history.

Table 6.1

Bleeding	Pain	Uterus	Cardiovascular system	Fetus	Mother
Slight	Mild	Irritable	Unchanged	Unaffected	Well
Moderate	Moderate/labour	Labour	Compensation	Distressed	Distressed
Severe	Severe/labour	Hard/labour	Compensation/decompensation	Death	Shocked

Mild bleeding

- Admit and observe after instituting general procedures.
- If the mother is in labour and the fetus is mature, rupture the membranes to check the state of liquor and provide access to the fetus for direct fetal heart rate monitoring.
- Close observation is mandatory. This includes extended cardiotocography if conservative management is adopted. Further placental separation can occur.

Moderate bleeding

- Replace blood loss.
- Carry out coagulation screen and correct defects.
- Rupture the membranes, administer oxytocics if labour is delayed.
- Perform caesarean section for fetal distress. Coagulation defects must first be excluded.
- An indwelling drain for the abdomen and wound after caesarean section is advised.
- An experienced obstetrician and anaesthetist are required.
- Ensure strict fluid balance and monitor the renal output (>20 ml/h).
- Epidural anaesthesia is contraindicated if the mother is hypotensive or there is evidence of coagulopathy.
- Presence of pre-eclampsia requires close watch for blood pressure fluctuations, renal shut down and electrolyte disturbances. These mothers are best observed on labour ward until clinically stable.
- Keep uterus contracted by intravenous syntocinon infusion after delivery.
- A neonatologist must attend delivery. Fetal blood loss (asphyxia pallida) will require urgent resuscitation.

Severe bleeding (See 'Major obstetric haemorrhage' above)

- Fetal death is usual. The aim is to resuscitate and evacuate the uterus.
- Correct coagulation defects.
- Blood transfusion is required.

- Control fluid replacement by use of a central line (exclude coagulopathy).
- Rupture the membranes and encourage labour.
- Watch closely for blood pressure changes and onset of coagulopathy.
- Labour usually supervenes or follows syntocinon infusion. If not, caesarean section is justified if condition is stable, the cervix is unfavourable and there is no coagulation defect. Delay allows further decompensation of the situation and risks onset of coagulopathy.
- Keep uterus contracted after delivery to prevent risk of postpartum haemorrhage. The Couvelaire uterus may not contract well.

Placenta praevia

- This describes a placenta inserted partially or wholly in the lower uterine segment.
- Characteristically presents with unprovoked painless bleeding. Occasionally, bleeding may be provoked by sexual intercourse. Note evidence of uterine activity.
- It is discovered following clinical or ultrasound examination. Unstable lie or high presenting part at term should alert to this condition.

Grading of placenta praevia

- I The placenta is in the lower uterine segment but the placental edge does not reach the internal os.
- II The lower edge of the placenta reaches but does not cover the internal os.
- III The placenta covers the internal os asymmetrically.
- IV The placenta covers the internal os symmetrically.

Grading is not clinically useful for predicting severity of antepartum haemorrhage.

Management

Management depends upon the gestational age, the amount of blood loss, fetal position and the placental site (in cases of minor placenta praevia):

- Apply the general guidelines for antepartum haemorrhage.
- Consider expectant management if the gestational age is less than 37 weeks when bleeding is mild. Close observation is mandatory.
- It is safer to consider tocolytics in cases of antepartum haemorrhage due to uterine activity and placenta praevia.
- Ensure cross-matched blood is available at all times.
- For moderate bleeding after 36 completed weeks or if bleeding is severe or continues after 24 weeks, caesarean section should be performed. Additional cross-matched blood must be available. A senior obstetrician and anaesthetist should be available to assist or advise especially where placentation is anterior.
- Remember placenta accreta in an anterior placenta with a previous caesarean section scar.
- Examination in theatre is acceptable when diagnosis is uncertain or when there is a grade I anterior placenta praevia (see Box 6.2).

Fits

Pregnancy can aggravate an existing tendency to fits (epilepsy) or convulsions can complicate pre-eclampsia (eclampsia). The presence of hypertension, proteinuria and generalized oedema and past history of epilepsy are important points that need to be considered in this situation.

Two-thirds of cases of eclampsia occur before and a third after delivery, sometimes 3 or more days post partum (12%).

Eclampsia

Guidelines for management

- Stop/prevent fitting. Give intravenous magnesium sulphate (4 g over 15 min).
- Reduce blood pressure. Give hydralazine/labetalol/nifedipine (care should be taken when combining magnesium sulphate and nifedipine; this combination is best avoided (calcium chelator and calcium blocker)). Both

---

Box 6.2   Examination in theatre

Requirements
- Blood must be available in theatre.
- No fetal distress.
- Prepare mother for caesarean section.
- Lithotomy position.
- Palpate around fornices. An interposing placenta will distance presenting parts.
- Locate the cervix and examine with a single digit in enlarging circles. The placenta has a spongy feel.
- Brisk bleeding indicates the need for immediate delivery.

For grade I anterior placenta praevia, rupture the membranes and attempt vaginal delivery. Close surveillance is mandatory. All other grades of placenta praevia necessitate caesarean section.

---

drugs can have a synergistic effect which can cause significant hypotension.
- Anticipate complications. Review mother frequently and monitor closely in a high dependency unit with senior staff involvement.
- Deliver the baby. Consider induction of labour or caesarean section. A major complication is fetal or maternal mortality.

Magnesium sulphate

- This drug is used for seizure prophylaxis. This is the current drug of choice in eclampsia (dispensed in 50% w/v solution with 1 g in 2 ml).
- There must be a protocol for magnesium sulphate administration.
- After the loading dose (4–5 g given slowly over 15–20 min) infuse 1–2 g/h for maintenance (20 ml Mg SO_4 in 250 ml normal saline at 50 ml/h.
- Infusion should be continued for 24 hours. Ensure tendon reflex is present, note urine output (should be 30 ml/h or 100 ml/4 h).
- The first sign of toxicity is loss of the knee reflex.
- Calcium gluconate 10% intravenously is given as antidote (require 10–20 ml).
- Continuous monitoring of O_2 saturation is required.
- Magnesium sulphate increases sensitivity to muscle relaxants (non-depolarizing).

Fluid balance

- Insert an indwelling urinary catheter and keep a strict input/output chart with hourly running totals.
- Total fluid intake should not exceed 2.5 l over 24 hours. Colloids can be used with caution for fluid challenges (200 ml) if the urine output is decreased.

Box 6.3   Hydralazine treatment

Mode of action
- Direct acting vasodilator
- Can cause sodium and fluid retention
- Plasma half-life 2–3 hours.

Contraindications
- Known hypersensitivity
- Systemic lupus erythematosus
- Tachycardia
- High output state (thyrotoxicosis)
- Aortic or mitral stenosis
- Isolated right ventricular failure due to pulmonary hypertension.

Cautions
- Renal impairment
- Ischaemic heart disease
- Surgery can exaggerate hypertension.

Side effects
- Tachycardia, palpitations, flushing hypotension, anginal symptoms, oedema, heart failure
- Headache, dizziness, peripheral neuritis
- Arthralgia rash
- Proteinuria, increased plasma creatinine, haematuria, renal failure
- Gastrointestinal disturbances, abnormal liver function
- Agitation, anxiety
- Dyspnoea.

Compatibility
Incompatible with dextrose.

Acute treatment
5 mg by slow (1 mg/min) intravenous bolus
Check blood pressure (BP) every 5 minutes for 30 minutes, or until BP is stable at <100 mm/Hg diastolic, then every 15 minutes for further 60 minutes.

Maintenance
40 mg hydralazine in 40 ml 0.9% saline (via syringe pump) giving 1000 micrograms/ml solution
Start at 40 micrograms/min (2.4 ml/h)
At 30 min 80 micrograms/min (4.8 ml/h)
At 60 min 120 micrograms/min (7.2 ml/h)
At 90 min 160 micrograms/min (9.6 ml/h)
Do not increase if pulse is >140 or if target BP is reached. Reduction by 10–20 microgram/min every 30 minutes.

- Frusemide is used for pulmonary oedema in the presence of over hydration, particularly with heart failure or with impending renal failure.

Antihypertensives
See Boxes 6.3 and 6.4.

Suspected fetal death

Any mother presenting with diminished fetal movements must be examined at once.

- Check for fetal heart rate.
- Reassure mother if the fetal heart is heard. Obtain a 30 minute external cardiotocographic trace of the fetal heart for inspection.
- Discharge for home if the antenatal history suggests no cause for concern. Admit and investigate if obstetric complications are present.

Box 6.4   Labetalol treatment

Cautions
- Asthma
- Heart failure
- Cardiogenic shock
- Arterial-ventricular block.

Side effects
- Postural hypotension
- Tiredness, weakness, headache, rashes, scalp tingling
- Difficulty in micturition
- Epigastric pain
- Nausea, vomiting
- Rarely lichenoid rash.

Oral therapy
200 mg oral loading then 200 mg oral tds
Increase to a maximum of 600 mg qds.

Intravenous therapy
- Acute: bolus dose for acute therapy, 5–10 mg IV slowly (5–10 min), effective within 5 minutes and lasts for 6 hours
- IVI solution: 5 mg/ml (200 mg in 40 ml).

Set a target BP. Increase infusion as stated until target BP is reached.

Start at 20 mg/h (= 4 ml/h)
At 30 min 40 mg/h
At 60 min 80 mg/h
At 90 min 160 mg/h

To reduce, decrease by 10 mg/h every 30 min as required. Convert to oral therapy by giving 200 mg orally 1 h prior to stopping infusion, followed by 200 mg tds.

- Perform ultrasound scan if fetal heart is not heard. If fetal death is confirmed by ultrasound scan findings to double check, inform the mother and partner immediately. Transfer to a quiet room for natural expression of grief. Discuss openly possible reasons for the tragedy but protect from any feeling of guilt.
- At a convenient time discuss the proposed course of further action.
- Suppress lactation.
- A post-mortem examination should be requested (negotiate level of examination).
- Request an X-ray examination if indicated.
- Provide a follow-up appointment for further counselling.

Cardiac arrest and cardiopulmonary resuscitation (CPR) in the obstetric mother

Cardiac arrest in late pregnancy or during delivery is a rare event. It usually accompanies major complications (e.g. amniotic fluid embolism). The physiological changes in late pregnancy often hamper effective cardiopulmonary efforts.

Some causes include:

- total spinal anaesthetic
- local anaesthetic toxicity from unintentional intravascular injection
- trauma
- pulmonary embolism
- amniotic fluid embolism.

Physiological changes in pregnancy relevant to cardiopulmonary resuscitation are:

- mothers become hypoxic more readily (20% decrease in their functional residual capacity and 20% increase in their resting oxygen consumption)
- the enlarged uterus can decrease compliance during controlled ventilation
- aortocaval compression in the supine position necessitates lateral tilt.

Procedure

- Tilt the uterus to the left side. A member of the team should be instructed to act as a 'human wedge' by kneeling down (both knees). Mother is placed across the wedge of the bent knees.
- CPR should begin immediately after ensuring airway. Follow advanced cardiac life support programme.
- If CPR is not successful after 5 minutes, caesarean delivery must be performed.
- CPR should be continued throughout the procedure.

REFERENCES

Caspi E, Lotan Y, Schreyer P 1983 Prolapse of the cord: reduction of perinatal mortality by bladder instillation and caesarean section. Israel Journal of Medical Sciences 19: 541–545
Chetty R M, Moodley J 1980 Umbilical cord prolapse. South African Medical Journal 57: 128–129

Vago T 1970 Prolapse of the umbilical cord. A method of management. American Journal of Obstetrics and Gynecology 107: 967–969

7

Normal labour and delivery

D. Liu, P. M. Thwaites

MYOMETRIAL ACTIVITY – PREGNANCY

During pregnancy the uterus is usually in a quiescent state. In the third trimester mothers experience low amplitude, poorly synchronized Braxton Hicks or practice contractions. Substances which contribute to inhibit myometrial activity include progesterone from placental syncytiotrophoblast and chorion; myometrial parathyroid hormone-related peptide; nitric oxide and relaxin from the myometrium, decidua, chorion and amnion in addition to prostacyclins. The process of myometrial contraction requires activation of calmodulin, a calcium binding protein with calcium ions, which then in turn activates the enzyme myosin light chain kinase to produce adenosine triphosphate; this powers actin and myosin filaments to slide over each other to produce shortening. Inhibitors of myometrial activity act by increasing intracellular levels of cyclic nucleotides to prevent release of calcium ions from intracellular stores or by reducing myosin light chain kinase activity.

Towards term a number of processes occur which predispose to activation or preparation of the myometrium for onset of labour. Formation of gap junctions by increases in contraction-associated proteins such as connexin-43 enhance cell-to-cell coupling. Receptors for oxytocin and stimulatory prostaglandins are also increased. These changes are associated with myometrial stretch when the uterus enlarges and with the higher levels of oestrogens derived partly from placental conversion of fetal dehydroepiandrosterone (DHEAS) where they also exert a local oestrogen effect. In addition to increased DHEAS production, activation of the fetal hypothalamic–pituitary adrenal axis in late pregnancy results in more fetal cortisol biosynthesis. Fetal cortisol competes to reduce the local progesterone effect and stimulate synthesis of corticotropin-releasing hormone from the placenta and fetal membranes for production of prostaglandins by the latter structures.

MYOMETRIAL ACTIVITY – LABOUR

Initiation of labour remains unclear but prostaglandins are implicated in myometrial contraction. Isoforms of phospholipase A_2 or C, activated by varying requirements for calcium ions, liberate arachidonic acids from membrane phospholipids. Prostaglandin synthase in amnion and chorion convert arachidonic acids to primary prostaglandins. For prostaglandin E_2 (PGE_2) there are four main receptor subtypes labelled EP-1–EP-4. These receptors are distributed in the myometrium in varying concentrations. Stimulation of EP-1 and EP-3 results in contractions whilst stimulation of the other two receptors leads to relaxation. These, together with corticotrophin-releasing hormone related cyclic adenosine monophosphate (AMP) in the lower uterine segment, contribute to fundal dominance.

Onset of labour is associated with a substantial increased myometrial sensitivity to oxytocin stimulation and a three- to five-fold increase in oxytocin production by chorio-decidual tissue. Oxytocin raises concentrations of free calcium in the myocytes to promote myometrial contraction.

Fetal membranes covering the internal cervical os exhibit a decreased production of the 15-hydroxyprostaglandin dehydrogenase enzyme which metabolizes prostaglandins. More local prostaglandin production is available for cervical effacement and dilatation. This effect is supplemented by release of collagenase through increased cytokine activity.

Onset of labour is most likely between midnight and 0500 hours when maternal secretion of oxytocin peaks and the myometrium is most sensitive to oxytocin and prostaglandin.

These changes in steroid and protein concentrations return to non-pregnant levels 48–72 hours post partum.

Uterine work

Myometrial contraction exerts pull in circular and longitudinal directions (Fig. 7.1). The term fundal dominance is used to describe travel of myometrial contractions from the fundus of the uterus towards the cervix. The starting point or pace maker for myometrial activity is situated near the point of insertion of the fallopian tubes into the uterus. The spread of myoelectrical activity through the uterus requires 1 minute. Approximately another minute is needed for adequate relaxation. Blood vessels must traverse the myometrium to reach the placenta. Contractions occurring more than once every 2 minutes contribute to poor myometrial relaxation and reduce blood and hence oxygen supply to the fetus. When two contractions are noted every 10 minutes for an hour consider possible onset of labour. In established labour contraction rates range between 3 and 5 per 10 minutes.

In early labour the uterus is not working at maximum capacity. This may be because the number of myometrial cells contracting is limited, or contraction is poorly synchronized or of short duration. As labour progresses contraction becomes more efficient and uterine work increases. Capacity for work cannot, however,

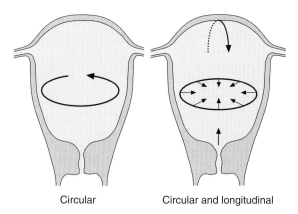

Circular   Circular and longitudinal

Figure 7.1 Myometrial contraction exerts pull in circular and longitudinal directions.

increase indefinitely. A stable phase for ability to work results once maximal work output is achieved for the individual mother. When the stable phase (Fig. 7.2a) is achieved additional stimulation by oxytocics is of little value and can be harmful. Uterine work has been expressed:

- classically as Montevideo units which are intensity (mmHg) times number of contractions per 10 minutes. The intensity is taken as the height reached by the recorded contraction from the resting tone (Fig. 7.2b).
- as kilopascals per 15 minutes, included as a display in contemporary models of fetal monitors when intrauterine transducers are used. The range for normal labour is 700–1500 kilopascals per 15 minutes.

Intrauterine pressure (IUP)

The viscoelastic myometrium always exerts a pressure on the amniotic fluid. This resting pressure or tone is usually 6–12 mmHg. Amniotic fluid is not compressible.

Measurement is achieved by:

- Insertion of a fluid-filled polythene tube into the uterine cavity. This tube is connected to a transducer capable of measuring changes in hydrostatic pressure.
- Insertion of a catheter-tipped pressure transducer into the uterine cavity (Fig. 7.3). This is a more costly but simpler system.
- Palpation and external (tocometers) assessment do not indicate IUP.

Intensity of uterine contractions increases throughout pregnancy. Towards term pressures up to 30 mmHg may be recorded. During labour intrauterine pressure increases to levels of 60–80 mmHg. Contractions of this intensity are still detectable for 48 hours post partum but the frequency diminishes after 12 hours.

General comments

- Normal efficient uterine activity is associated with fundal dominance and regular

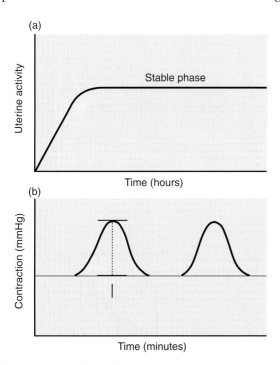

Figure 7.2 (a) Graph of uterine activity with stable phase (plateau) for individual mother. (b) Montevideo unit = intensity (amplitude of recorded contraction) × contractions per 10 minutes. The Alexandra unit, a refinement, takes into consideration duration of the contraction.

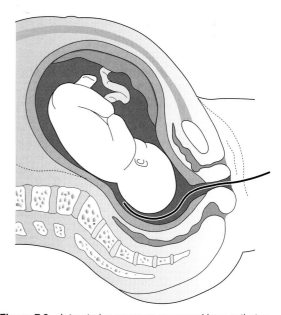

Figure 7.3 Intrauterine pressure measured by a catheter-tipped pressure transducer placed above presenting part is less affected by mother's movement.

synchronized contractions of good (more than 40 mmHg) intensity.

- Contractions should last between 40 and 60 seconds with an adequate interval in between when intrauterine pressure can return to resting tone.
- Uterine contractions are more efficient when the mother lies on her side.
- Primiparous labour is generally associated with contractions of greater intensity than those in multiparae.
- Early amniotomy shortens labour with no detrimental effect on fetal outcome nor an increase in assisted delivery. In uncomplicated labours, mother's preference must be considered. The increased uterine activity of labour exerts an additional pressure on the amniotic fluid. Measurement of this intrauterine hydrostatic pressure (IUP) indicates the strength of the contraction.
- Epidural analgesia may lengthen both first and second stage of labour, and increases incidence of fetal malposition and vaginal instrumental delivery (incidence reduced by routine oxytocin).

Effect of uterine activity on the cervix

Before labour

In the weeks before labour that portion of the uterus between the internal os and the reflection of the uterovesical fold of the peritoneum is attenuated by stretch and Braxton Hicks contractions to form the lower segment. This allows the presenting part of the fetus, particularly in primiparous mothers, to settle or engage into the pelvis.

In labour

Labour is traditionally divided into two stages:

- First stage – onset of labour to full cervical dilatation. This includes the latent and active phases of labour.
- Second stage – full dilatation to delivery of the baby. The duration approximates 60 minutes in primiparous and 30 minutes in multiparous

mothers. Management/intervention should not be based solely on these suggested times. A little more time can be allocated to avoid unwelcome interference if both the fetus and the mother are well. On the other hand with complications or fetal distress, elective assisted delivery or a shortened second stage is advised.

Effacement precedes cervical dilatation. Initially uterine activity is expanded to achieve effacement. This period, the latent phase of labour, takes on average 9 ± 6 hours in the primiparous and 5 ± 4 hours in the multiparous mother. The cervix is usually up to 2 cm dilated when labour begins. At the end of the latent phase cervical dilatation is usually between 3 and 4 cm. Once effaced further uterine activity produces rapid cervical dilatation of at least 1 cm per hour in both parous and nulliparous mothers. This, the active phase of labour, takes on average 6 hours to reach full cervical dilatation (Fig. 7.4). Multiparous mothers approach labour with more cervical effacement hence a shorter latent phase and thus a shorter labour.

It is common practice to plot the rate of cervical dilatation to indicate the progress of labour. This is usually charted on a single sheet of paper designed for recording labour events over a 24 hour period. Provision is also made for registering fetal heart rate (every 30 minutes), uterine contractions (every 30 minutes), rate of head descent and medication. Cervical dilatation detected by vaginal examination is recorded every 2–4 hours. This graphic representation of

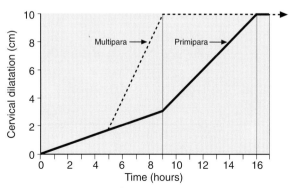

Figure 7.4 Partogram. Primipara and multipara showing latent phase and steep active phase to full cervical dilatation.

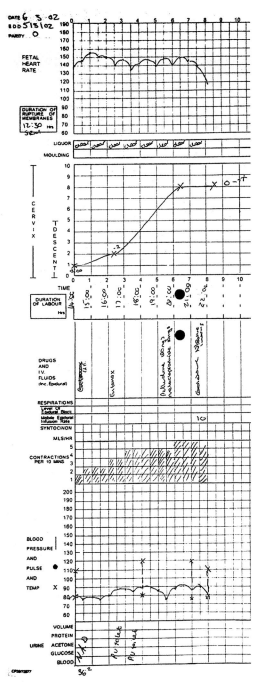

Figure 7.5 Example of a partogram in use showing a concise summary of events in labour.

parturition (partogram) summarizes and depicts, visually, the events in labour (Fig. 7.5). Cervical dilatation lagging 2–3 hours behind that expected from the normal graph (Fig. 7.6) should suggest to medical attendants the need for reassessment.

Effect of uterine activity on the fetus

- Blood vessels traversing the myometrium to supply the placenta and fetus are compressed during uterine contractions. Delivery of nutrients and, particularly, oxygen is impeded or curtailed once the intrauterine pressure exceeds 40 mmHg. Increased myometrial tension or tone and rapid recurring contractions further reduce the capacity to supply the fetus and hence threaten hypoxic insult.
- Compaction or curling up of the fetus occurs with each contraction. Pressure is exerted on the presenting parts, such as the fetal head. During passage through the birth canal the whole fetus is compressed and this can evoke vagal stimuli.
- The substantial increase in fetal catocholamine production helps switch off fetal lung liquid production.
- The fetus is gradually expelled into the vagina in the process of birth.

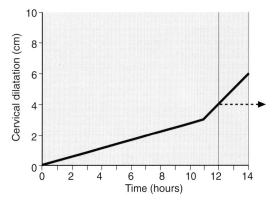

Figure 7.6 Partogram showing deviation (—) from the expected course.

The mechanism of labour is illustrated in Box 7.1.

Management of the delivery

Position

The squatting posture is well suited to delivery. A mother adopting the lithotomy position propped up with pillow and her legs drawn back essentially achieves this posture but has the added advantage of allowing attendant access to assist delivery.

Aseptic conditions

Gloves and gown are mandatory for the attendant conducting the delivery. The mother should be

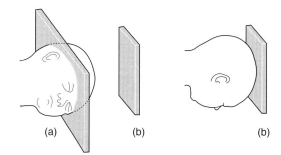

(a) (b) (b)

Figure 7.7 The widest part of the inlet (a) (transverse diameter) and outlet (b) (anteroposterior diameter) is represented geometrically. Fetal head enters in the occipito transverse then rotates to address anteroposterior diameter of outlet.

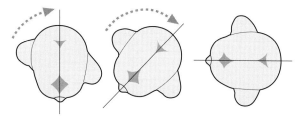

Figure 7.8 Delivery of the head by extension.

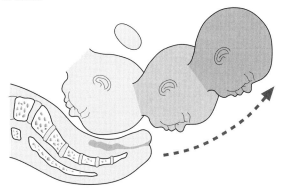

Figure 7.9 Restitution showing the relationship of the sagittal axis of fetal head to allow delivery of shoulders in the anteroposterior diameter of the pelvic outlet.

Box 7.1 Mechanism of labour

Flexion and entry
Uterine contractions cause further flexion and entry of the fetal head into the pelvis, usually in the occipito transverse (Fig. 7.7).

Descent and internal rotation
Descent occurs to the level of the ischial spines when levator ani muscles assist internal rotation to align the sagittal sutures for delivery through the widest anteroposterior diameter of the outlet.

Extension and delivery of the head
Distension of the lower part of the vagina evokes reflexes which stimulate the urge to push. Pushing is achieved by the valsalva response and contraction of diaphragmatic and abdominal muscles. The head stretches the vagina and vulva as it delivers. Extension occurs once the head passes beneath the symphysis pubis. Fetal membranes usually rupture before this stage (shown in sequence in Fig. 7.8).

Restitution, external rotation and delivery of the shoulders
The head rotates to occipito lateral or restitutes to align naturally perpendicular to the shoulders. The shoulders, having entered the pelvis in the oblique diameter, rotate so the bisacromial diameter of the shoulder delivers in the anteroposterior diameter of the pelvic outlet. Further rotation of the head laterally accompanies rotation of the shoulders (Fig. 7.9).

Delivery of the body
The shoulders deliver assisted by lateral flexion of the body. Once this is achieved the rest of the fetus delivers readily as the uterus contracts down (Fig. 7.10).

---

draped and the vulval area cleansed. Deliver onto sterile towels.

Medical attendant

The medical attendant is usually stationed on the mother's right. Place the left hand on the fetal head as it 'crowns' (passage of the biparietal eminences through the vulva) to maintain flexion and prevent expulsive delivery.

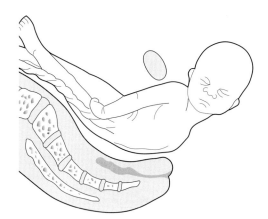

Figure 7.10 Delivery of the body by lateral flexion.

The right hand is used to guard the perineum and cover the anus with a sanitary pad. If necessary assist extension of the fetal head by lifting the chin. Consider if an episiotomy is required.

Delivery of the head

Instruct the mother to pant once the head is crowned. This prevents forceful pushing and repeated gentle increase in intra-abdominal pressure created by panting nudges the head out. Aspirate the mouth then the nose of the baby at the first opportunity. Give intramuscularly 0.5–1 ml of syntometrine to the mother (a combination of the synthetic oxytocic syntocinon 5 units per ml and ergometrine maleate 0.5 mg per ml). The oxytocic effect is evident in $2^1/_2$ (syntocinon) to 7 minutes (ergometrine). It assists uterine contraction, placental separation and thereby controls blood loss. For mothers at risk of haemorrhage, give ergometrine intravenously (oxytocic effect in 1 minute).

Delivery of the shoulders

Once external rotation is completed, direct the head gently downwards to assist delivery of the shoulders. When the anterior shoulder appears beneath the symphysis insert a finger into the anterior axilla and lift the body upwards watching

the perineum at the same time to avoid extension of the episiotomy or tearing of the perineum.

Umbilical cord

Cut the cord within 1 minute of birth. This interval allows additional transfusion of more than one-third of the fetal blood volume. Do not wait for cessation of pulsation as the placenta may be separated and fetal exsanguination can result. Free any loose cord around the neck over the head or shoulders and proceed with the delivery. If the cord is tight around the neck or fetal resuscitation is anticipated clamp and cut the cord at once and deliver the baby.

Management of the third stage

The third stage is the interval between delivery of the fetus and delivery of the placenta. Placental separation is shown by:

- a lengthening of the cut cord
- a show of blood
- elevation of the fundus as the uterus contracts following separation of the placenta.

Delivery of the placenta

The placenta usually separates within 3 minutes and is delivered within 5 minutes after birth. Proceed as follows.

- Stand on the mother's right side. The uterus should be contracted.
- The left hand is placed suprapubically. Straddle the uterus with the thumb on one side and the rest of the fingers on the other for better control (Fig. 7.11). Press backwards towards the mother to align the uterus with the vaginal axis. Figure 7.12 shows straightening of the uterus.
- Grasp cord with the right hand and apply gentle traction in line with the pelvic axis (approximately 45° to the horizontal). If the cord springs back once pressure is removed, placental separation is not complete. Wait. If the placenta is separated, controlled traction will deliver the placenta (Fig. 7.13).

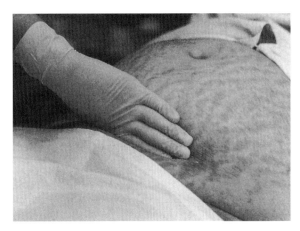

Figure 7.11 Placement of the hand for delivery of the placenta.

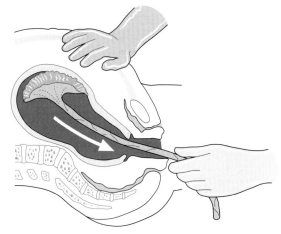

Figure 7.13 Controlled cord traction facilitates delivery of the separated placenta.

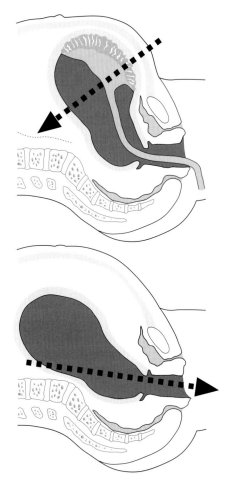

Figure 7.12 Alignment of uterus with vaginal axis assists the delivery of the placenta.

- Rotate the placenta to wind the membranes into a cord to assist their complete delivery.
- Inspect the placenta, the membranes and the cord for abnormalities and completeness.

Effect of uterine activity on the mother

Management guidelines

- Labour evokes feelings of anxiety and anticipation particularly in the primipara, where labour is lengthy and when complications are present. Emphasize teachings from antenatal classes and offer support.
- Pain threshold varies with individuals. Ensure comfort and avoid distress (see Box 7.2).
- Nurse the mother on her side or in a semi-reclining position (semi-Fowler) to assist labour and avoid compression of the inferior vena cava. Flexibility in attitude of the attendants is needed to accommodate individual preferences (check birth plans).
- Maintain energy requirements and electrolyte balance.
- Record the pulse, blood pressure and temperature at regular intervals.
- Special precautions are required if there is preexisting maternal medical disease or complications (for example, supplementary hydrocortisone to cover stress of labour).

Box 7.2 Administration of Entonox

- Check that gas cylinders are not empty and that they have been stored at room temperature. The two gases may separate if stored at low temperatures (−7°C).
- Ensure the mask fits over the nose and mouth with no air leaks from the sides of the mask.
- Analgesia begins at 20 seconds and is maximum at 45 seconds. The interval between onset of uterine contractions and sensation of pain is 20–30 seconds in the latent phase and 10–15 seconds in the active phase of labour. Use the mask at the beginning of contractions for the maximum analgesic effect at the height of the contraction.
- Instruct the mother to inhale deeply through the mouth and exhale rapidly to make the machine

click. The gas mixture is only released from the demand valve in the machine when the mother inhales deeply.
- If the mother is particularly sensitive to nitrous oxide use the mask only when contractions become uncomfortable.
- For analgesia in the second stage, time contractions and breath 30 seconds before each contraction. Instruct the mother to take two to three quick deep breaths on the mask during a contraction prior to her pushing efforts.
- The mother must be instructed to hold the mask herself. Should she become anaesthetized the mask will fall away from her face and allow recovery.

- Good communication and documentation is essential particularly when there is digression from standard practice.

FURTHER READING

Grammatopoulos D K, Hillhouse E W 1999 Role of corticotrophin-releasing hormone in onset of labour. Lancet 354: 1546–1549

Howell C J, Kidd C, Roberts W et al 2001 A randomised controlled trial of epidural compared with non-epidural analgesia in labour. British Journal of Obstetrics and Gynaecology 108: 27–33

Lye S J, Ou C W, Teoh T G et al 1998 The molecular basis of labour and tocolysis. Feto-Maternal Medical Review 10: 121–136

Patel F A, Clifton V L, Chawalisz K et al 1999 Steroidal regulation of prostaglandin dehydrogenase activity and expression in human term placenta and chorio decidua in relation to labour. Journal of Clinical Endocrinology and Metabolism 84: 291–299

Petraglia F, Florio P, Nappi C et al 1996 Peptide signalling in human placenta and membranes: autocrine, paracrine, and endocrine mechanisms. Endocrine Review 17: 156–186

Sangha R K, Walton J C, Ensor C M et al 1994 Immunohistochemical localisation, mRNA abundance, and activity of 15-hydroxyprostaglandin dehydrogenase in placenta and fetal membranes during term and preterm labour. Journal of Clinical Endocrinology and Metabolism 78: 982–989

Sparey C, Robson S C, Bailey J et al 1999 The differential expression of myometrial connexin-43, cyclooxygenase-1 and -2 and Gsa proteins in the upper and lower segments of the human uterus during pregnancy and labour. Journal of Clinical Endocrinology and Metabolism 84: 1705–1710

Steer P J, Carter M C, Gordon A J et al 1978 The use of catheter-tip pressure transducers for the measurement of intrauterine pressure in labour. British Journal of Obstetrics and Gynaecology 85: 561

UK Amniotomy Group 1994 A multi-centre randomised trial comparing routine versus delayed amniotomy in spontaneous first labour at term. British Journal of Obstetrics and Gynaecology 101: 307–309

8

Intrapartum nutrition and electrolytes

P. Tomlinson

Pregnant women approach labour with a mild degree of respiratory alkalosis and metabolic acidosis. Their capacity to utilize glucose is reduced. Defects in energy requirements are often met by increased lipolysis. This causes a small rise in plasma ketone levels throughout pregnancy. Ketonuria, however, is not observed unless plasma ketone concentration rises above 6–8 mmol/l. Gluconeogenesis does occur in the fetal liver and kidneys, but the main glucose supply is from the mother. This is provided by diffusion, across the placenta, down a concentration gradient. Fetal blood glucose levels are one-third to one-half that of the mother. As a result, fetal glucose rises and falls with changes in maternal nutritional state, and maternal starvation will reduce fetal plasma glucose. In labour, the fetal glucose requirement is 7–10 mg/kg/min. Water diffuses freely across the placenta. Sodium and chloride concentrations are similar in maternal and fetal plasma, but potassium levels are higher in fetal than maternal blood, 6.4 mmol/l and 4.6 mmol/l respectively. The likely mechanism of this is an active transport system.

CHANGES IN LABOUR

Labour further affects maternal metabolism and plasma electrolytes. Also, certain modern therapeutic measures employed in the management of specific problems in labour produce additional changes. The basic factors involved are:

1. The energy of labour is provided predominantly by glucose, and most women enter

labour with little reserve for sustained aerobic metabolism. Moderate accumulation of lactate causes a fall in maternal plasma pH to 7.34 and a fall in $PaCO_2$ to 4–4.5 kPa.

2. Oral intake of food and water is often discouraged to reduce the risk of regurgitation of stomach contents and aspiration pneumonia (Mendelson's syndrome). This can occur in association with general anaesthesia, and abrupt changes in levels of conciousness produced by acute major pathology in labour or by use of heavy sedation.

3. Exertion, stress, and prolonged or high dose use (>16 mU/min syntocinon) of intravenous oxytocics enhance antidiuretic hormone (ADH) production. This produces water retention and hyponatraemia.

4. In a bid to avoid sodium retention, electrolyte free dextrose solutions are commonly used to maintain hydration and to temporarily expand the vascular compartment when epidural analgesia is commenced. This practice can, however, cause hyponatraemia in the fetus and the mother. Rapid falls of plasma sodium to <128 mmol/l may produce cerebral oedema, confusion, convulsions, coma and even death.

5. Beta-sympathomimetics, such as salbutamol, are often used intravenously for reducing the risk of preterm labour. These drugs encourage migration of potassium into cells, producing hypokalaemia. There is an additional ADH effect and possible hyperglycaemia due to their sympathetic activity.

6. Vomiting due to pain, stress or opioids and altered renal function due to complications such as pre-eclampsia (PET) can further contribute to water and electrolyte imbalance.

NUTRITION IN LABOUR

Controversy

Some obstetricians and midwives now believe that in the absence of risk factors that could lead to operative delivery of the baby (perhaps with the aid of general anaesthesia), or serious intra-partum morbidity (e.g. PET), strict limitations of oral intake in labour to small amounts of water could be relaxed (Michael et al 1991). Frye even claims that eating in labour allows women to feel normal and healthy (Frye 1994). Their main argument, however, is that ingestion of adequate quantities of calories and water orally prevents significant acidosis and electrolyte disorder. Most protagonists of oral feeding in labour cite studies demonstrating that administration of clear fluids up to 2 hours before elective surgery does not increase gastric volume or acidity in non-pregnant patients, providing that they do not consume solid food (Kallar & Everett 1993).

Applying the results of such studies to mothers in labour may be ill-advised:

1. The interval between the last full meal and the onset of labour varies a great deal between patients. Ultrasound examination will often demonstrate that two-thirds of pregnant mothers have solid gastric contents regardless of the time elapsed since their last meal (Kallar & Everett 1993).

2. Systemic administration of opioids to mothers in labour dramatically delays gastric emptying (Nimmo et al 1975). Epidural or spinal local anaesthetic/opioid mixtures may produce similar effects though not all studies agree on this.

3. Mothers in labour may require caesarean section or other life saving interventions at any time. The interval between last oral intake and induction of anaesthesia could be substantially within 2 hours.

It is appropriate, therefore, to continue the practice of restricting oral intake in labour, probably to 60 ml/h water or other non-particulate fluid in uncomplicated labours until further research clarifies this issue.

Management guidelines

Uncomplicated/spontaneous labour

- Assess condition after admission.
- Restrict oral intake to clear fluid.
- Prescribe opiates and antiemetics.
- Monitor fluid balance.

Complicated labour: where fetal compromise/operative delivery more likely

- Assess condition after admission.
- Restrict oral intake to <60 ml/h water.
- Set up intravenous infusion: this should include 69 g glucose/m^2/24 h to avoid ketonuria.
- Strict fluid balance chart.
- Regular urine checks for ketones.
- Regular plasma electrolyte checks.

KEY POINTS

- Nutrition in labour, especially in presence of complications, is important but requires much regular attention to detail.
- Opioid administration by any route may cause significant delays in gastric emptying.
- Mothers in labour who have not received appreciable quantities of parenteral opioid may be allowed up to 60 ml/h clear fluid to drink.

REFERENCES

Frye A 1994 Nourishing the mother. Midwifery Today 31(Autumn): 25–26

Kallar S K, Everett L L 1993 Potential risks and preventive measures for pulmonary aspiration: new concepts in preoperative fasting guidelines. Anaesthesia and Analgesia 77: 171–182

Michael S, Reilly C S, Caunt J A 1991 Policies for oral intake during labour: a survey of maternity units in England and Wales. Anaesthesia 46: 1071–1073

Nimmo W S, Wilson J, Prescott L F 1975 Narcotic analgesics and delayed gastric emptying during labour. Lancet 1: 890–893

9

Analgesia and anaesthesia

D. M. Levy

Obstetric *analgesia* is the diminution of pain in labour; *anaesthesia* is the abolition of sufficient sensation to allow operative delivery.

The experience of pain represents a complex combination of physiological, psychological, emotional and conditioned responses. Modern regional blocks can relieve pain in labour whilst preserving some sensation of uterine contractions and the ability to push. If forceps or caesarean section become necessary, it is possible to produce surgical anaesthesia rapidly by extension of the block. In the vast majority of cases general anaesthesia can be avoided. General anaesthesia is nowadays reserved largely for those cases where a regional block is either contraindicated or has failed.

ANALGESIA FOR LABOUR

Inhalational analgesia

Sixty to seventy per cent of labouring mothers in the UK seek to achieve analgesia by inhalation of a 50:50 mixture of nitrous oxide and oxygen (N_2O/O_2). Marketed as Entonox and Equanox the gas mixture is supplied in cylinders with blue body and blue/white shoulders and is piped to delivery rooms in many hospitals.

The gas is self-administered by inspiration through a facemask or mouthpiece, which opens a demand valve. Diffusion from alveoli to pulmonary capillaries and delivery to the brain by the cardiac output is not instantaneous – inhalation should start as soon as a contraction begins, in order that maximum effect is achieved at its peak.

The drug is non-cumulative, and doesn't affect the fetus. N_2O/O_2 causes sedation, which is highly variable amongst mothers. Some appear to be dreaming or drunk; others become somnolent or even briefly unrousable. Hyperventilation with N_2O/O_2 can be followed by a short period of apnoea. The mother should hold the mouthpiece or mask herself. If she loses consciousness, she will let go. A few breaths of air eliminate the N_2O and consciousness will invariably be regained soon.

A number of studies have questioned the analgesic effect of N_2O/O_2. Pain is still perceived under the influence of the drug – it is merely rendered more bearable by the intoxicated state.

The risk of cross-contamination between mothers sharing breathing systems dictates that mouthpieces and masks should be disposable, or sterilized between use. Either a new disposable breathing system should be used for each mother, or a disposable breathing system filter interposed between the tubing and mouthpiece/mask.

Parenteral opioids

Clinical studies of pain scores have cast doubt on the analgesic efficacy of opioids in labour. The drugs are certainly sedative, inducing a feeling of disorientation, and thereby making pain more tolerable.

All opioids can induce maternal and neonatal respiratory depression (decreased Apgar and neurobehavioural scores). Gastric emptying is inhibited, and the incidence of nausea and vomiting increased.

Midwives can prescribe and administer controlled drugs in accordance with locally agreed policies and procedures. In the UK, pethidine is the most widely used intramuscular (IM) opioid. A usual dose of 100 mg lasts around 3 hours. Plasma pethidine concentrations are maximal in the neonate when the mother has received the drug about 3 hours before delivery. It is therefore illogical to withhold the drug if delivery is imminent, for fear of causing neonatal respiratory depression.

Naloxone is a specific opioid antagonist. The neonatal dose is 10 micrograms.kg^{-1} IM, repeated if necessary.

Comparisons of diamorphine 5 mg, meptazinol 100 mg and tramadol 100 mg with pethidine 100 mg have failed to demonstrate any convincing benefits.

An antiemetic (e.g. cyclizine 50 mg or prochlorperazine 12.5 mg) should be given IM along with whatever the chosen opioid. Because of the additive risk of respiratory depression, IM opioids should never be given in the event of inadequate regional analgesia without prior reassessment of the mother by an anaesthetist.

Transcutaneous electrical nerve stimulation (TENS)

Electrical impulses applied to the skin via flexible carbon electrodes from a battery-powered stimulator modulate the transmission of pain by closing a 'gate' in the dorsal horn of the spinal cord. The effect is similar to massage of the lower back by a birthing partner.

TENS is used in about 1 in 20 labours in the UK. The technique is completely free from adverse effects, and can diminish the need for other analgesic interventions.

A study comparing TENS and 'sham TENS' (TENS devices which appeared to be working but had been disabled) failed to demonstrate reduced pain scores in labour. After delivery, however, those mothers who had had working TENS retrospectively rated their analgesia more highly. More of these mothers stated they would choose TENS again in a future labour.

Regional analgesia for labour

Regional analgesia is the provision of pain relief by blockade of sensory nerves as they enter the spinal cord. Local anaesthetic can be introduced into epidural or subarachnoid (intrathecal) spaces, or both.

The epidural space is identified by the loss of resistance to depression of a syringe plunger as a Tuohy needle is advanced (Fig. 9.1) through the ligamentum flavum. A catheter is then threaded

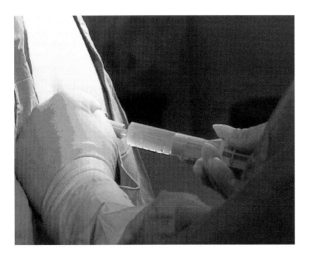

Figure 9.1 Advancement of Tuohy needle with loss of resistance to syringe plunger.

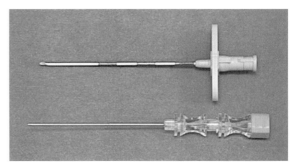

Figure 9.3 Epidural Tuohy (above) and spinal needles.

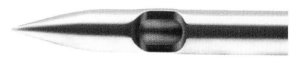

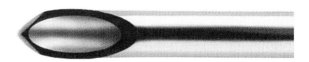

Figure 9.4 Pencil point (above) and cutting bevel tip spinal needles (courtesy of SIMS Portex Ltd).

through the Tuohy needle (Fig. 9.2) to facilitate top-ups or continuous infusion.

The subarachnoid space (containing cerebro-spinal fluid) is a few millimetres deeper, inside the meninges. Needles used for spinal injection are much finer than Tuohy needles (Fig. 9.3). A significant advance has been the development of 'pencil point' tips (Fig. 9.4). Compared to standard cutting bevel or Quincke needle tips, the leak of cerebrospinal fluid (CSF) and likelihood of consequent headache are vastly reduced.

A trained anaesthetist *must* always be immediately available wherever regional analgesia is provided. Regional techniques improperly administered can be as hazardous as any general anaesthetic.

The resources that should be available on every labour ward in the event of complications (see below) which might arise during the provision of regional analgesia are listed in Box 9.1.

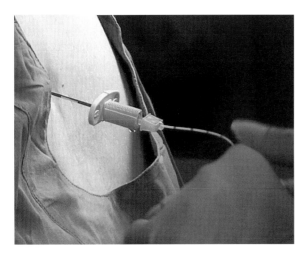

Figure 9.2 Tuohy needle advanced through ligamentum flavum, with catheter in epidural space.

Box 9.1 Resources for treatment of complications during the provision of regional analgesia

- laryngoscope and blades
- tracheal tubes and stylettes
- oxygen source
- suction source with tubing and catheters
- self-inflating bag and mask for positive pressure ventilation
- drugs – vasoconstrictor (e.g. ephedrine), anaesthetic induction agent (e.g. thiopental), neuromuscular blocking drug (e.g. succinylcholine)

Compared with every other analgesic technique, pain relief from regional blockade is undoubtedly superior. Ninety per cent of consultant obstetric units in the UK provide a 24-hour epidural service; the average epidural rate is 24%.

Since blockade of motor fibres causes relaxation of pelvic floor muscles and impairs expulsive efforts, provision of adequate maternal analgesia with as little motor block as possible has emerged as a goal common to all regimens. Intermittent epidural boluses, continuous epidural infusions, and patient controlled epidural analgesia (PCEA) all provide comparable pain relief and maternal satisfaction.

Unlike local anaesthetics, which prevent conduction of nerve impulses, opioids act on specific receptors in the spinal cord. Synergistic mixtures of local anaesthetic and opioids (usually fentanyl) have permitted significant reductions in the amount of local anaesthetic used.

Side effects specific to the use of opioids are respiratory depression (in the most unlikely event that opioid spreads cephalad to reach the brainstem) and pruritus.

Combined spinal–epidural analgesia entails an initial subarachnoid injection of fentanyl mixed with a tiny amount of local anaesthetic. The resulting motor block is sufficiently minimal for mothers to retain enough muscle power to walk around in labour. However, proprioception (information from joint receptors to maintain balance) can be impaired. In the absence of any proven advantage to mother or baby of walking in labour, some argue that it is hard to justify the risk of falling.

Signed consent is not necessary for regional analgesia in labour. Verbal consent is sufficient, and a brief record should be made in the notes of the risks/benefits that have been discussed.

Table 9.1 outlines contraindications to regional analgesia, together with the associated risks.

A full blood count (FBC) is not required unless antepartum bleeding has occurred, anaemia is suspected, or there is evidence of pre-eclampsia. If the platelet count is normal, a coagulation screen is not necessary. If a pre-eclamptic mother's overall condition is deteriorating an FBC should have been processed no more than 2 hours before

Table 9.1 Contraindications to regional analgesia, with associated risks

Contraindication	Risk
Uncorrected anticoagulation or coagulopathy	Vertebral canal haematoma
Local or systemic sepsis (pyrexia >38°C not treated with antibiotics)	Vertebral canal abscess
Hypovolaemia or active haemorrhage	Cardiovascular collapse secondary to sympathetic blockade
Maternal refusal	Legal action
Lack of sufficient trained midwives for continuous care and monitoring of mother and fetus for the duration of epidural blockade	Maternal collapse, convulsion, respiratory arrest; fetal compromise

a regional block is undertaken. If platelet count is $70–100 \times 10^9 \, l^{-1}$ or if the trend is steadily downwards, a coagulation screen must be normal if spinal/epidural block is to be undertaken. Petechiae or platelet count $<70 \times 10^9 \, l^{-1}$ are indications for platelet transfusion. Aspirin therapy alone is not a contraindication to regional analgesia.

Low molecular weight heparins (LMWH) pose the risk of vertebral canal haematoma and consequent spinal cord or nerve root compression. This risk has to be weighed against the risk of emergency general anaesthesia in a mother denied regional blockade. As far as possible, institution of regional blocks – and removal of epidural catheters – should be undertaken when anti-factor Xa activity is least. After delivery, continued vigilance for signs of haematoma is essential. If symptoms of leg weakness or numbness, back pain, or bowel/bladder dysfunction develop (onset can be delayed beyond 24 hours) neurological/neurosurgical advice should be sought without delay.

Whilst vertebral canal haematoma or abscess are exceedingly rare, transient neuropathy has an incidence of about 1 in 2000. Mothers can be reassured that epidural analgesia does *not* cause new, long-term backache.

All mothers should be warned about the possibility of dural tap – the inadvertent tearing of the meninges by Tuohy needle or epidural catheter, which should have an incidence of <1%. This complication can predispose to two potentially serious sequelae – total spinal anaesthesia, and post-dural puncture headache (PDPH). The majority of those who develop PDPH will require an epidural 'blood patch'.

Other points worthy of explanation before performing a regional block in labour are listed in Box 9.2.

The rate of cervical dilatation, duration of second stage and instrumental delivery rate are similar when epidural analgesia is established before or after 4 cm cervical dilatation.

Regional analgesia does not result in an increase in the overall caesarean section rate or the specific rates for dystocia or fetal distress. However, a significant proportion of those mothers who undergo caesarean section for dystocia will have had epidural analgesia for labour. *Risk factors for dystocia produce painful labour and a desire for epidural analgesia.*

It is well worth explaining in advance to mothers with risk factors for operative delivery that *analgesia* for labour can be converted to effective *anaesthesia* to facilitate forceps or caesarean delivery. Many mothers need time to consider the notion of being awake for a caesarean section. Hurried explanations of anaesthetic options while mothers are being wheeled to theatre predispose to demands for general anaesthesia.

The two principal potential complications of epidural injection of local anaesthetic are *local anaesthetic toxicity* and *total spinal anaesthesia*. Aspirating the catheter to exclude intravenous or subarachnoid placement can prevent both. The delivery of local anaesthetic to the brain and heart by the bloodstream causes the symptoms and signs of toxicity (Table 9.2).

Epidural venous engorgement in a pregnant mother predisposes to blood vessel puncture in up to 1 in 5 epidurals. If blood is aspirated, flush with saline and withdraw catheter by another 1 cm. If blood is still present, resite at another interspace. Local anaesthetic toxicity is not an issue with spinals because the mass of drug injected is so much smaller.

Total spinal anaesthesia is the effect of excessive local anaesthetic within the subarachnoid space.

Box 9.2

Before starting a regional block in labour inform mothers about:
- potential failure to site catheter or achieve perfect analgesia
- necessity to resite catheter in 5–15% of procedures
- localized backache for about 48 hours due to bruising.

Epidural analgesia is *associated* with the following:
- longer first and second stages of labour
- maternal pyrexia (>38°C)
- increased incidence of fetal malposition
- increased use of oxytocin
- increased incidence of instrumental vaginal deliveries.

Table 9.2 Symptoms and signs of local anaesthetic toxicity

Symptoms	Signs
Numbness of tongue or lips	Slurring of speech
Tinnitus	Drowsiness
Light-headedness	Convulsions
Anxiety	Cardiorespiratory arrest

If a dose intended for the epidural space is inadvertently delivered to the subarachnoid space, cephalad spread can cause respiratory arrest by blocking innervation of the diaphragm (C3,4,5), and profound hypotension secondary to extensive sympathetic blockade.

A 'total spinal' can occur even when no CSF has been apparent on aspiration, and remains a possibility hours after initiation of an epidural block and following several top-ups. The risk of inadvertent subarachnoid block is not eliminated by epidural catheterization at another interspace after the dura has been punctured, because the dural tear might still allow passage of local anaesthetic to the CSF.

In addition to local anaesthetic toxicity and total spinal anaesthesia, maternal collapse can occur as a result of:

- Massive haemorrhage (which might be intrauterine or intraperitoneal)
- Amniotic fluid embolism (anaphylactoid syndrome of pregnancy)

- Pulmonary thrombo-embolism
- Eclampsia
- Intracranial haemorrhage
- Myocardial infarction.

The management of collapse in a pregnant mother is detailed in Box 9.3.

Attendants should also:

- make sure they know where the resuscitation equipment and emergency drugs are kept
- keep up to date with the latest UK Resuscitation Council algorithms.

Establishing regional analgesia – practical points

- The mother's cooperation must be secured to maximize the chances of success. Consider fentanyl 50 micrograms intravenously for the mother unable to keep still on account of intense pain. Particularly in multiparous mothers, it is worth checking that sudden escalation of pain is not indicative of imminent delivery or uterine rupture.
- Secure IV access (14 g or 16 g cannula) must be established using local anaesthesia. An IV crystalloid infusion must be started, although a fluid bolus is not required unless the mother is evidently dehydrated.
- Meticulous aseptic precautions are essential, with gown, gloves, hat and mask.

- Loss of resistance to saline is associated with a lower incidence of dural tap and patchy block compared with air. In the event of dubiety as to the origin of fluid appearing at the hub of a Tuohy needle, CSF and saline can be distinguished on the criteria detailed in Table 9.3.
- The epidural drug regimen used in two Nottingham teaching hospitals is detailed in Box 9.4.
- A bilateral block to the sensation of cold (ice or ethyl chloride spray) to T10 should relieve the pain of uterine contractions. If a block rises above T6 (Fig. 9.5) the infusion should be stopped, and restarted at a lower rate when the block height has regressed to T10.
- If maternal systolic blood pressure falls below 75% of baseline (e.g. from 120 to 90 mmHg), administer O_2, turn on side, raise legs and give 500 ml fluid rapidly. If blood pressure remains low, ephedrine 3–10 mg IV should be given in preference to more fluid.
- Light diet is acceptable for mothers without obstetric risk factors.
- Any neurological deficit persisting >6 hours after the last top-up or discontinuation of an infusion should be referred for a neurological opinion.

Table 9.3 Distinction between CSF and saline

	CSF	Saline
Temperature	warm	cold
Protein	present	absent
Glucose	at least a trace	absent
pH	≥7.5	<7.5

Box 9.3 Collapse in the pregnant mother

- Call for help.
- Clear the airway.
- Administer high flow oxygen (10 l/min) by facemask.
- If apnoeic, ventilate with bag and mask. Apply cricoid pressure to occlude the oesophagus. Intubate the trachea as soon as is feasible.
- Relieve aortocaval compression by manual displacement of the uterus or wedging the right hip with pillows.
- If pulseless, start external cardiac compressions.
- *Delivery by caesarean section is indicated if there is no response to advanced life support within 5 minutes.*

Box 9.4 Drug regimen for epidural analgesia

- *Initial dose*: fentanyl 50 micrograms + bupivacaine 0.25% 10 ml given in two divided doses 5 minutes apart.
- *Subsequent infusion*: fentanyl 150 micrograms + bupivacaine 0.5% 10 ml + 0.9% saline to a total volume of 60 ml. Infuse at 5–15 ml/hour.
- *'Escape' top-up for inadequate analgesia*: bupivacaine 0.25% 5 ml, maximum of two doses/hour.

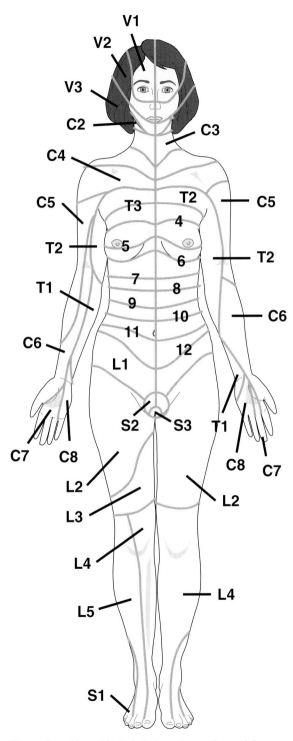

Figure 9.5 Map of (anterior) dermatomes (artwork by Rachel Ellaway© 2000 University of Edinburgh, with permission).

Initial management of dural tap

Either a Tuohy needle or a catheter can breach the meninges. In such cases follow the guidelines below:

- If CSF flows from the hub of the needle, thread catheter into the subarachnoid space. If CSF is aspirated from the catheter, leave catheter in subarachnoid space. Alternatively, resite the catheter at another interspace.
- If a catheter is used in the subarachnoid space, make sure that the filter is clearly labelled as *spinal*. Boluses of bupivacaine 0.25% 1–2 ml will provide excellent analgesia for labour. For caesarean section anaesthesia, titrate 0.5 ml increments of 0.5% hyperbaric bupivacaine.
- Subsequent headache might be averted by development of an inflammatory reaction around a catheter left at the site of the dural tear for a further 12 hours. The filter cap must be taped over and clearly labelled 'do not inject'.
- Only if headache develops during labour need elective forceps be advised at full dilatation. Caesarean section might be indicated in the rare instance of headache confining a mother to lying flat.
- There is no evidence that enforced postpartum recumbence will prevent development of PDPH. Ensure prescription of regular analgesia and a laxative such as ispaghula husk to prevent straining.

Epidural blood patch

This is indicated if *postural* headache or neckache persists beyond 24 hours. Note that the site of a headache is variable; the diagnostic feature is that it is worse after sitting up.

Procedure

- In theatre, with full aseptic precautions, the epidural space is identified at or below the original puncture site, and unless limited by back or leg pain (due to arachnoid irritation), up to 20 ml of the mother's freshly aspirated blood is slowly injected.

- After lying flat for 1–2 hours, the mother can mobilize cautiously. Around one in five mothers require a subsequent procedure.
- If headache is of insufficient severity to necessitate blood patch and the mother is discharged, arrangements must be made for review in the community. If her symptoms are not resolving within the next week, she should be readmitted. Chronic CSF leakage is not a benign condition – intracranial subdural haematoma is a rare complication of the reduced CSF pressure.

Pudendal block

This provides anaesthesia for episiotomy/perineal repair and low forceps delivery. Both pudendal nerves are blocked as they pass under and slightly posterior to the ischial spines (see Ch. 11). Use of lidocaine 0.5% allows injection of a generous total volume (up to 40 ml). If epidural analgesia has been established during labour, pudendal block will be unnecessary. A top-up of bupivacaine 0.5% with the mother sitting (in order that the local anaesthetic might bathe the sacral nerve roots) will provide excellent anaesthesia.

ANAESTHESIA FOR CAESAREAN SECTION

Preoperative preparation

Protracted deprivation of food and oral fluid should be avoided. Elective caesarean section cases should no longer be instructed to be 'nil by mouth' from midnight. An appropriate fasting policy is:

- last solid food 6 hours pre-theatre
- last cup of squash or tea/coffee (with semi-skimmed, not full-fat milk) 2 hours pre-theatre
- unrestricted *sips* of *water* until operation.

Mothers scheduled for elective caesarean section should receive the following antacid prophylaxis because of the tiny risk of pulmonary aspiration of gastric contents in the course of general anaesthesia after failed regional block (and the remote possibility of high spinal anaesthesia causing inability to protect the airway):

- Two oral doses of ranitidine 150 mg, approximately 8 hours apart.
- 30 ml 0.3 M sodium citrate immediately before transfer to theatre.
- Mothers in labour with significant risk factors for caesarean section should have oral ranitidine 150 mg 8-hourly.

Results of a recent FBC and blood group/antibody screen should be available. A haemoglobin concentration of 8–10 g.dl^{-1} should not normally be an indication for preoperative transfusion, but a check should be made that serum has been saved by the laboratory in case a cross-match becomes necessary.

Urea and electrolytes are requested only if specifically indicated.

Non-elective cases

- *Only about 10% of emergency caesarean sections are totally unpredictable.* Anaesthetists, obstetricians and midwives should discuss those mothers whose babies have prior evidence of compromise (e.g. intrauterine growth restriction [IUGR], or poor biophysical profiles/umbilical artery Doppler studies).
- Unless a senior obstetrician is certain that vacuum extraction/outlet forceps delivery will succeed, regional blockade should be sufficient to facilitate immediate caesarean section, should it prove necessary.
- When a decision to proceed to caesarean section is made for a mother labouring with an epidural, it is important to be clear how long the obstetrician is prepared to wait for surgical anaesthesia. Placental abruption, uterine scar dehiscence, sudden persistent fetal bradycardia and cord prolapse are indications for *immediate* caesarean section (not necessarily under general anaesthesia for all mothers). Dystocia ('failure to progress') should allow plenty of time for topping up an epidural.
- Mothers needing emergency surgery should be transferred in left lateral position, with

syntocinon discontinued. All mothers should be positioned on the table with 15° left lateral tilt.

- Monitoring of electrocardiogram, non-invasive blood pressure and pulse oximeter is essential for all mothers. For general anaesthesia, capnography (CO_2 monitoring) is vital to confirm tracheal intubation. Inhalational agent monitoring will aid prevention of awareness. Suction apparatus must be working and close to hand.

Causes of maternal mortality directly attributed to anaesthesia over the last few decades, along with deaths *associated with* anaesthesia, are listed in Box 9.5.

Spinal anaesthesia

Spinal anaesthesia has become the most common technique for elective caesarean section, on account of its speed and efficacy compared with epidural anaesthesia. Placental blood flow is maintained provided that hypotension is avoided. The possibility of having to resort to general anaesthesia should always be discussed, and the airway evaluated preoperatively.

Box 9.5   Maternal mortality attributable to and associated with anaesthesia

Causes of maternal mortality attributable to anaesthesia
- Pulmonary aspiration of gastric contents
- Failed tracheal intubation (and reintubation)
- Airway obstruction from neck haematoma
- Anaphylaxis to induction/neuromuscular blocking drugs
- Regional block without IV access
- Inadequate antagonism of neuromuscular block
- Excessive local anaesthetic with clonidine in a combined spinal–epidural.

Deaths associated with anaesthesia 1994–1996
- Pulmonary hypertension plus cardiac failure
- Amniotic fluid embolism
- Eclampsia/pre-eclampsia
- Haemorrhage
- Sepsis
- Phaeochromocytoma
- Mitral valve disease.

Only rarely should pressure of time preclude institution of a spinal block for a mother who has been labouring without epidural analgesia.

Establishing spinal anaesthesia – practical points

- Avoid aortocaval compression at all times.
- Atropine (0.6 mg) and ephedrine (30 mg diluted to 3 mg.ml^{-1}) should be drawn up, with drugs for general anaesthesia readily available.
- Establish IV infusion (14 or 16 g cannula).
- All drugs for subarachnoid injection must be drawn up through a particulate filter.
- **Hyperbaric** (heavy) **bupivacaine 0.5% 2.5 ml** is appropriate for most mothers. Mothers with preterm pregnancies have a requirement for more local anaesthetic compared to those at term, probably because of reduced caval compression and displacement of the dura by engorged epidural veins.
- Preservative-free **morphine 0.1 mg** mixed with the local anaesthetic will provide prolonged postoperative analgesia in conjunction with regular paracetamol and non-steroidal anti-inflammatory drugs (NSAIDs) unless contraindicated (see section on postoperative analgesia).
- Infuse a litre of Hartmann's or 0.9% saline rapidly. Maintain systolic arterial pressure above 100 mmHg by administration of IV boluses of ephedrine 3 mg.
- Hypotension with tachycardia (heart rate >100) is best treated with 50–100 microgram increments of phenylephrine, which tends to increase blood pressure with concomitant decrease in heart rate. *Phenylephrine must be diluted to 100 microgram/ml before use.*
- *Anaesthesia* (inability to appreciate light touch) should extend to T4 (see Fig. 9.5) at the time of delivery. A block to cold from the sacral segments to T4 should be confirmed and documented before surgery starts. Because spinal anaesthesia virtually guarantees complete sensory loss below the most cephalad level, the lower dermatomes do not need to be tested.
- In the event of an inadequate block, a second intrathecal injection should not be administered,

because it is difficult to estimate an appropriate safe dose. If time permits, site an epidural catheter and top up cautiously with bupivacaine 0.5%. If delivery is urgent, general anaesthesia will be indicated.

Epidural anaesthesia

This is most often used when epidural *analgesia* has been established during labour.

Indications

- There are very few occasions when a mother with a working epidural in labour should need general anaesthesia for caesarean section on the grounds of lack of available time to establish surgical anaesthesia.
- Epidural anaesthesia is indicated in certain clinical conditions (e.g. congenital heart disease) when a regional technique is preferable to general anaesthesia but spinal anaesthesia is relatively contraindicated because of its potential for sudden sympathetic blockade.
- Epidural anaesthesia might be favoured when provision of optimal postoperative analgesia by infusion of bupivacaine/fentanyl in a high dependency area is warranted, e.g. severe pre-eclampsia.

Establishing epidural anaesthesia – practical points

- The top-up to achieve surgical anaesthesia should be administered in theatre with full monitoring attached, rather than in the delivery room.
- Bupivacaine 0.5% (plain) 15–20 ml works as fast and as reliably as any other solution for transformation of low-dose epidural analgesia into surgical anaesthesia. Note that about 7 times as much local anaesthetic is required for an equivalent effect from drug administered into the epidural as opposed to subarachnoid spaces.
- Opioids both improve the quality of the block during surgery (e.g. when the uterus is exteriorized) and provide postoperative anal-

gesia in conjunction with an NSAID. Epidural fentanyl in labour does not preclude a further perioperative dose of up to 100 micrograms (e.g. 50 micrograms during establishment of the block and a further 50 micrograms after delivery). The subsequent epidural administration of diamorphine 2.5 mg will provide excellent postoperative analgesia.

- Epidural anaesthesia may leave normal sensation in the most caudal (sacral) dermatomes. Block of the sacral roots is important to prevent pain during traction and pressure on the vagina. All dermatomes from S5–T4 (Fig. 9.5) should be tested to cold on both sides, and the upper and lower limits of the block (and any missed segments) documented.
- Intra-operative pain is more likely with epidurals than spinals. Intravenous alfentanil in 0.5 mg increments can be used to control breakthrough pain, and should not be withheld for fear of neonatal respiratory depression. 0.25% isoflurane in 50% oxygen/50% nitrous oxide administered by anaesthetic breathing system is also effective. Unrelieved, persistent pain must be managed with general anaesthesia.

Combined spinal–epidural anaesthesia

- The initial subarachnoid injection can be deliberately conservative, to reduce the risk of a dangerously high block (e.g. in the morbidly obese, or mothers with difficult airways). In addition, the haemodynamic consequences of spinal anaesthesia will be minimized.
- The subarachnoid block can be augmented by subsequent epidural top-ups (particularly useful if protracted surgery is anticipated).
- The epidural catheter can be used in the postoperative period (e.g. severe pre-eclampsia).

General anaesthesia

With good antenatal education and preoperative explanation of the benefits of regional anaesthesia, few mothers should insist upon general anaesthesia.

Mothers should be fully assessed wherever possible before transfer to theatre. Pre-oxygenation and cricoid pressure should be explained, and the airway assessed.

Practical points

- The anaesthetic machine and equipment for management of difficulty with airway establishment, e.g. McCoy laryngoscope, gum elastic bougie, laryngeal mask airway (LMA), and cricothyrotomy device, must be checked. *Never reach for an unfamiliar device for the first time in a crisis!*
- A dedicated trained assistant must be available to apply pressure on the cricoid cartilage, to occlude the oesophagus.
- Site a 14 g or 16 g cannula in the hand or wrist with Hartmann's solution or 0.9% saline running. Ensure establishment of left lateral tilt.
- Optimize head and neck position for intubation. In addition to left lateral tilt, a slight head-up position should offer some protection against gastro-oesophageal reflux.
- Pre-oxygenate via a close-fitting facemask for 3 minutes or until the end tidal oxygen concentration approaches 90%.
- Administer a precalculated bolus of thiopental 5–7 $mg.kg^{-1}$ or etomidate 0.3 $mg.kg^{-1}$. Give succinylcholine 100 mg or rocuronium 0.6 $mg.kg^{-1}$ and instruct assistant to apply cricoid pressure.
- In the event of failure to intubate the trachea, maintain cricoid pressure and attempt to ventilate the lungs with 100% oxygen via facemask. If ventilation proves impossible, release cricoid pressure (which might be causing airway obstruction). Regurgitation and pulmonary aspiration of gastric contents is neither inevitable nor necessarily fatal.
- An LMA can restore airway patency by displacing the tongue, epiglottis, or larynx from the posterior pharyngeal wall. Again, any increased risk of regurgitation compared with a tracheal tube is of secondary importance to establishing oxygenation. If recovery from suxamethonium has occurred, surgery can proceed with spontaneous respiration of vapour in 100% O_2.

- Mechanical ventilation should be instituted after successful tracheal intubation or placement of an LMA when a non-depolarizing neuromuscular blocker has been used. Check for continued pulmonary inflation and adjust minute volume to maintain end tidal CO_2 at around 4.0 kPa.
- With the airway secured and recovery from succinylcholine block confirmed, give increments of a non-depolarizing relaxant, e.g. atracurium 25 mg or rocuronium 30 mg, guided by the response to peripheral nerve stimulation. *Smaller doses will be required in the presence of therapeutic serum magnesium concentrations.*
- Adjust fresh gas mixture to 33–50% O_2 in N_2O with at least 1.0 minimum alveolar concentration (MAC) (inspired) of isoflurane or sevoflurane. If low fresh gas flows are used in a circle system, be guided by end tidal vapour and N_2O concentrations.
- Concerns about the effects of anaesthetic agents on the newborn baby and uterine tone have been overemphasized in the past. Excessively light general anaesthesia risks awareness and has a detrimental effect on uteroplacental blood flow.
- After the cord is clamped, give IV morphine 10–20 mg. Do not discontinue inhalational anaesthesia until surgery has been completed.
- Reverse neuromuscular block using a peripheral nerve stimulator to confirm full recovery.

Tocolysis and oxytocics

On occasions, uterine relaxation might be requested to facilitate procedures such as delivery of a second twin.

Practical points

- IV increments of glyceryl trinitrate (GTN) **50 micrograms** are effective. Hypotension does not seem to occur in mothers already venodilated by a regional block. GTN can alternatively be given by metered dose (400 micrograms) sublingual spray.
- Syntocinon 5 units should be given by slow IV bolus at every caesarean section as soon as

the cord has been clamped (the last cord if multiple pregnancy). This dose can be repeated. Syntocinon can cause transient vasodilatation, hypotension and tachycardia, but is effectively treated with IV increments of phenylephrine 50 micrograms.

- The requirement for a Syntocinon infusion (40 units over 6 hours) can be anticipated in certain cases. Mothers with a distended uterine cavity after multiple pregnancy or a macrosomic baby, and those who have had a prolonged labour, antepartum haemorrhage or placenta praevia are at risk of postpartum haemorrhage.
- Avoid the large unnecessary fluid load of successive 500 ml bags of Syntocinon (with its antidiuretic effect) in 5% dextrose by using small diluent volumes administered by syringe pump.

POSTOPERATIVE ANALGESIA

- Unless contraindicated, **diclofenac** 100 mg suppository should be administered at the end of surgery. Prescribe *regular* diclofenac, 50 mg 8-hourly plus **paracetamol** 1 g 4–6-hourly, max 4 g/24 h oral or per rectum. **Dihydrocodeine** 30–60 mg orally, 4-hourly (max 240 mg/24 h) is prescribed 'as required'.
  Contraindications to diclofenac (and other NSAIDs) are listed in Box 9.6.
- Because of the risk of respiratory depression, it makes sense to restrict *parenteral* administration of opioids for at least 6 hours after spinal or epidural fentanyl and 12 hours after

---

Box 9.6 Contraindications to diclofenac

- Hypovolaemia or continuing bleeding (risk of renal hypoperfusion).
- Pre-existing renal impairment (including poor urine output in pre-eclampsia). If diclofenac is withheld, reconsider prescription once oliguria has resolved.
- Asthma with history of sensitivity to NSAIDs (can prescribe if mother has previously taken other NSAIDs without adverse effects).
- Peptic ulceration.
- Hypersensitivity to NSAIDs.

---

morphine or diamorphine. Following general anaesthesia, titrate morphine intravenously. For postnatal analgesia, prescribe morphine 10–15 mg IM 3-hourly 'as required' *or* 1 mg boluses (5 min lockout) via patient controlled analgesia system (PCAS).

- Ensure low molecular weight heparin (LMWH) has been prescribed *(pulmonary embolism is the leading cause of maternal death in the UK)*.
- Discharge to the ward only when cardiovascular and respiratory variables are acceptable and stable. Mothers must not be left alone in single rooms. Monitoring of respiratory rate, sedation, pulse and blood pressure must be charted in accordance with the unit's protocol.

PLACENTA PRAEVIA

The anaesthetist should engage in discussion with the obstetrician regarding the placental site and how much bleeding is anticipated. The risk of major haemorrhage is significantly increased if a previous caesarean section has been performed and the placenta is adherent to the myometrium (placenta accreta).

Practical points

- Regional anaesthesia is not necessarily contraindicated. However, the mother should be made aware that significant blood loss might ensue, and that being awake while large quantities of blood are rapidly infused might not be a pleasant experience. In the event of serious difficulty securing haemostasis, general anaesthesia might become desirable.
- Ensure that at least 4 units of red cells are available. Two IV lines (14 or 16 g cannulae) should be established with rapid fluid infusion devices primed. *Senior obstetricians and anaesthetists should be present in theatre.*
- Because the lower segment does not contract as effectively as the upper segment, there is a risk of postpartum haemorrhage after caesarean section for placenta praevia. Close postoperative monitoring and a Syntocinon infusion for at least 6 hours are essential.

PRE-ASSESSMENT

All units should have a referral system between obstetricians and obstetric anaesthetists. Trainees providing out-of-hours cover should never be presented with complex cases 'out of the blue'. Consider anaesthetic referral for any mother referred to a specialist physician's clinic (e.g. cardiology).

Anaesthetists' principal concerns are:

- the feasibility of epidural/spinal block – which depend on flexion of the lumbar spine and normal blood coagulation
- whether tracheal intubation at emergency caesarean section might be hazardous, e.g. because of limited neck flexion/mouth opening
- the influence of medical conditions and their treatment on the safe conduct of regional or general anaesthesia.

Criteria for referral are listed in Box 9.7.

PRE-ECLAMPSIA

Anaesthetists' contributions include provision of analgesia, blood pressure control, intravenous fluid/blood product administration and physiological monitoring.

Practical points

- Regional analgesia is strongly indicated to eliminate the pain and stress of labour and thus prevent further rises in blood pressure and improve uteroplacental blood flow. A regional block should not be regarded as a first-line treatment for hypertension – a loading dose of magnesium sulphate or specific antihypertensive agent should be administered first.
- Spinal anaesthesia does not cause excessive hypotension (the hypertension of pre-eclampsia is mediated humorally, not neurally by the sympathetic nervous system). Intravenous ephedrine boluses (3–6 mg) do not cause an exaggerated hypertensive response.

Box 9.7 Criteria for antenatal anaesthetic referral

Cardiovascular problems
- Congenital heart disease
- Valvular heart disease
- Arrhythmias
- Cardiomyopathy
- Poorly controlled hypertension

Respiratory problems
- Severe asthma (requiring steroids or hospital admission)
- Breathlessness which limits daily activity
- Cystic fibrosis, or any other chronic chest disease

Neurological/musculoskeletal problems
- Any back surgery e.g. laminectomy, surgery for scoliosis (rods may have been inserted)
- Congenital conditions, e.g. spina bifida
- Muscular dystrophy, myotonia
- Myasthenia gravis
- Demyelinating disease (multiple sclerosis)
- Spinal cord injury
- Rheumatoid arthritis or any condition affecting neck/jaw
- Cerebrovascular disease (e.g. aneurysm, arteriovenous malformation)

Haematological problems
- Anticoagulation
- Blood clotting/platelet disorders
- Mothers who have been treated for malignancy (e.g. lymphoma, leukaemia)

Airway problems
- Previous difficulty with intubation
- Inability to open mouth or move jaw or head normally

Drug-related problems
- Cholinesterase abnormalities – succinylcholine (Scoline) apnoea
- Allergy or adverse reaction to anaesthetic drugs
- Malignant hyperthermia
- Drug abuse

Other problems
- Morbid obesity – body mass index (weight ÷ height squared) >40 $kg.m^{-2}$
- Needle phobia
- Panic attacks
- Any obscure eponymous syndrome that no one seems to have heard of which may pose problems if emergency anaesthesia is needed
- Any mothers with concerns regarding analgesia or anaesthesia (e.g. previous problems with inadequate epidural for labour, or pain/awareness during caesarean section)

- General anaesthesia is indicated if there is a coagulopathy or symptoms/signs of impending eclampsia. Specific problems include laryngeal oedema, which might necessitate a smaller tube.

- Prior communication with the neonatal paediatrician is essential in order that preparation can be made for antagonism of opioid or provision of ventilatory support.
- The induction regimen should protect the cerebral circulation from hypertensive surges. Have a low threshold for direct arterial pressure monitoring.
- Attenuate the pressor response to intubation with alfentanil 10 micrograms.kg^{-1} or remifentanil 2 micrograms.kg^{-1} (preceded by glycopyrrolate 0.4 mg to prevent bradycardia) prior to rapid sequence induction.
- In the presence of therapeutic serum concentrations of magnesium sulphate, use reduced doses of non-depolarizing drugs for maintenance of neuromuscular block (e.g. mivacurium 0.15 mg. kg^{-1}). A peripheral nerve stimulator is *essential* to monitor the degree of block.
- Before extubation, consider specific therapy (e.g. labetalol in 10–20 mg increments) to avert a dangerous pressor response.
- If a swollen larynx was evident at laryngoscopy or intubation was traumatic, be extremely wary of postextubation stridor.

ECLAMPSIA

Fits occurring in late pregnancy and labour should be regarded as eclamptic unless proven otherwise. Alternative diagnoses include epilepsy, amniotic fluid embolism (anaphylactoid syndrome of pregnancy), intracranial pathology (tumours, vascular malformations, haemorrhage), water intoxication, and local anaesthetic toxicity.

Practical points

- Maintain airway patency and give 100% oxygen. If a clear airway cannot be achieved with facemask and Guedel airway, summon skilled anaesthetic assistance and intubate the trachea. Use a generous dose of thiopental or propofol ideally with alfentanil to help obtund the pressor response. Avoid aortocaval compression, and attempt to prevent trauma to the mother and fetus.
- Most initial fits will be self-limiting. After the convulsion has terminated, examine the mother for signs of pulmonary aspiration (tachypnoea, crackles/wheeze), and institute SpO$_2$ monitoring. Ensure that the fetal heart rate is determined without delay. Signs of fetal compromise secondary to maternal hypoxaemia or placental abruption will signal the need for emergency caesarean section.
- Depending on the conditions of mother and fetus, a regional anaesthetic *may* be appropriate (a single fit is not a contraindication to a regional block).
- Postoperatively, all eclamptic mothers who have an emergency caesarean section under general anaesthesia should be transferred to an intensive care unit for a period of sedation and ventilation. Ideally, brain imaging should be performed *en route* in order to exclude intracranial haemorrhage and ascertain whether there is evidence of cerebral ischaemia.
- Treat as for a non-pregnant patient with brain injury/cerebral ischaemia. If neuromuscular block is used, arrange neurophysiological monitoring (e.g. cerebral function analysing monitor) in order that further seizure activity might be identified.

FURTHER READING

Burnstein R, Buckland R, Pickett J A 1999 A survey of epidural analgesia for labour in the United Kingdom. Anaesthesia 54: 634–640

Carroll D, Tramèr M, McQuay H et al 1997 Transcutaneous electrical nerve stimulation in labour pain: a systematic review. British Journal of Obstetrics and Gynaecology 104: 169–175

Department of Health 1998 Report on confidential enquiries into maternal deaths in the United Kingdom 1994–1996. HMSO, London

Elbourne D, Wiseman R A 2000 Types of intra-muscular opioids for maternal pain relief in labour (Cochrane Review). In: The Cochrane Library, Issue 1. Update Software, Oxford

Shibli K U, Russell I F 2000 A survey of anaesthetic techniques used for caesarean section in the UK in 1997. International Journal of Obstetric Anesthesia 9: 160–167

10

Intrapartum fetal surveillance

D. Liu, E. R. Buckley, T. Fay

Most babies deliver without problems. In complicated pregnancies however, birth can be a hazardous process for the fetus. Intrapartum surveillance by manually assessing contractions and listening (60 seconds) at intervals (15 minutes in first stage, 5 minutes in second stage) to check the fetal heart rate is a well established obstetric practice accepted for uncomplicated pregnancies. Electronic instrumentation has been introduced to facilitate continuous intrapartum fetal monitoring (when auscultation suggests abnormality, when there is evidence of or potential fetal compromise). The fetus signals potential compromise by:

- alterations in heart rate,
- the development of acidosis,
- the passage of meconium,
- the presence of excessive moulding
- excessive movements.

PHYSIOLOGY AND PATHOPHYSIOLOGY

The fetal cardiac output is controlled mainly by the heart rate rather than stroke volume. Cardiac output also varies with gestation. About 50% of the fetal cardiac output is directed to the low resistant placental circulation for oxygenation and nutrients. Flow rate in the umbilical vein is approximately 100 ml/kg/min. The following statements are relevant to understanding intrapartum fetal surveillance:

- Normal fetal heart rate (FHR) is between 110 and 160 beats per minute (BPM). Vagal response slows the rate, for example during fetal head or cord compression, whilst in a healthy fetus sympathetic response or catecholamine release following anaemia, hyperthermia, sepsis or hypoxia will produce tachycardia up to a maximum of 220 BPM.

- A fetus with an intact brain and myocardium exhibits FHR accelerations of 15 BPM for more than 15 seconds above baseline recordings in response to fetal movements, tactile or auditory stimulation.
- The healthy fetus exhibits an intrinsic baseline FHR variability of 5–25 BPM. A 'flat' or 'silent' pattern with <5 BPM variability for ≤40 minutes can indicate fetal inactivity or fetal 'sleep'.
- The fetus can improve myocardial oxygenation through a reflex compensatory mechanism or 'diving reflex' by slowing the heart rate during uterine diastolic. This mechanism can produce transient changes described as variable or late decelerations, which in some 50% may signal the likely presence of metabolic acidaemia (normal umbilical artery pH is 7.26 ± 0.08). Fetal blood sampling is required to differentiate between physiological and pathological heart rate responses.
- Umbilical vein compression causes a reflex vagal parasympathetic response and produces transient variable decelerations. Like late decelerations, persistent appearance of these patterns correlates with possible presence of fetal acidaemia.

FETAL HEART RATE (FHR) – BACKGROUND

Fetal heart rate can be recorded intermittently by auscultation with a Pinard stethoscope or electronically by a Doppler instrument. Doppler recordings rely on ultrasound registration of the Doppler shift to signal fetal heart rate. Continuous electronic FHR monitoring (Fig. 10.1) was introduced to provide uninterrupted intrapartum recordings. A fetal scalp electrode and intrauterine pressure recordings were used to provide the described classic patterns of transient fetal heart rate changes. Intrapartum pressure recording of

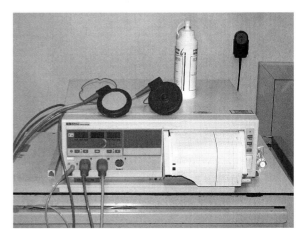

Figure 10.1 Example of machine used for continuous fetal heart monitoring.

uterine activity, however, is now usually replaced by use of external transducers to register sequential changes in uterine contraction. Correct placement of this external contraction device is important. Idiosyncrasies between the intrauterine and external methods for recording uterine contraction must be appreciated. The universal principle of need to understand the workings of tools used must apply since FHR change is read against the peak of the displayed uterine contraction.

Continuous electronic FHR monitoring is a screening adjunct for intrapartum fetal surveillance. Interpretation remains problematical and emphasizes need for constant education since failure to appreciate and react to signals of fetal insult is consistently identified as an avoidable factor in intrapartum fetal hypoxic damage or demise (DoH 1995). Contemporary recommendation is an ongoing programme of education for interpretation of FHR changes for all involved in intrapartum care (Maternal and Child Health Consortium 2000).

Screening fetal welfare by recording FHR changes (cardiotocograms – CTGs) should:

- Interpret changes against a set of accepted definitions (for example National Institute for Clinical Excellence 2001).
- Interpret against the clinical presentation and background.

Further points

- Drugs, e.g. pethidine, can blunt FHR responses, whilst procedures such as insertion of an epidural block, vomiting, catheterization and toileting can be followed by changes reflecting placental blood flow or vagal responses. Over 40% of fetuses in labour may show non-reassuring or abnormal traces. Discrepancy between fetal outcome, FHR and pH emphasizes that non-reassuring FHR changes should be interpreted as a need for review and/or check on fetal pH where appropriate. At best only 60–70% of pathological changes are indicative of fetal acidaemia.
- There is intra- and inter-observer variation in interpretation. Attempts to standardize interpretation are thwarted by lack of an internationally accepted guideline for interpretation and lack of consensus for terminology or definition.
- A tocodynamometer essentially only indicates presence of a contraction. The peak of uterine contraction registered by an external tocometer need not equate with recordings from an intrauterine catheter. The peak of the contraction using an external tocodynamometer (photo) varies with the site of placement on the mother's abdomen.
- There is no clear understanding of the relationship between FHR changes and fetal myocardial or cerebral oxygenation.
- A normal CTG pattern reassures that only 2% of babies will have a pH of <7.25 at birth.
- A well grown healthy fetus should withstand 90 minutes of hypoxic stress before the pH falls. Fetal reserve is less in a compromised fetus. The preterm fetus is more susceptible to hypoxia, particularly to damage of the Type II pneumocytes. There is, however, no means to indicate how much hypoxic insult a healthy fetus can withstand.
- In 90% of cerebral palsy the causative event occurs before onset of labour. In the remaining 10% intrapartum signs of hypoxia may reflect the presence of pregnancy compromise such as intrauterine growth restriction, fetal damage or infection.

- Usually hypoxaemia and metabolic acidaemia are progressive processes and timing of onset is difficult. Signs of fetal compromise are often insensitive and not specific to any particular cause.
- The fetus may be able to compensate until attendant effects of uterine contractions or strength of contractions produce added insult and threat of irreversible neurological damage.
- Fetal acidaemia may indicate ability of the fetus to respond appropriately to hypoxia. Metabolic acidaemia at birth is common (2%) and most of these babies do not develop neurological damage. Pathological acidaemia associated with increased risk of neurological damage is a pH <7.0 and a base deficit of >12 mmol/l. Existing fetal compromise must be kept in mind.
- The fetus is unlikely to be acidaemic if the fetal heart rate baseline is between 110 and 160 beats per minute, variability is within 5–25 beats per minute and there is no deceleration. Acidaemia is likely if there is bradycardia, no variability and persistent late or variable decelerations. In acute hypoxia the pH drops by 0.1 unit/minute.
- Fetal metabolic acidosis (pH <7.0 and base deficit of 12 mmol/l or more) is associated with increased risk of subsequent neurological deficit such as spastic quadriplegia.
- After 32 weeks the FHR patterns can be interpreted as for term babies. Before this gestation there are fewer accelerations, and decelerations of <20 seconds can occur spontaneously.
- Fetal sepsis is not usually associated with a low pH (pH <7.20) until the late stage of labour.
- A scalp electrode should not be used in mothers with the HIV or *Herpes simplex* virus. Do not attach clip to a fetus with a bleeding disorder, e.g. haemophilia.

FETAL HEART RATE – TYPES

During labour the fetal heart rate is described in terms of baseline rates (readings between contractions) and transient changes (readings during contractions). Four features (baseline rate, variability, presence of acceleration and deceleration) are used to assess fetal welfare.

Baseline fetal heart rate

Normal FHR is accepted as between 110 and 160 BPM recorded over 5 or 10 minutes.

Tachycardia, or FHR above 160 BPM, is known as the sympathetic or catecholamine response. It is severe if above 180 BPM. Causes include: maternal diseases such as infection and thyrotoxicosis; administered drugs, for example atropine, beta sympathomimetics and hydralazine; fetal infection and hypoxia. A rate of between 161 and 180 is non-reassuring.

Bradycardia is FHR below 110 BPM. Progressive or sudden slowing to less than 100 BPM suggests fetal decompensation. Causes include: known contribution by administered drugs such as opiates and local anaesthetics; fetal cardiac abnormalities, for example heart block; and fetal hypoxia. A rate between 100 and 109 is non-reassuring.

Baseline variability occurs when, as a consequence of a fixed stroke volume, the fetal heart rate speeds and slows to maintain a stable blood pressure and cardiac output. Normally this variability is >5–25 BPM (where 5 BPM is the distance between two faint horizontal score lines on recording paper). The term 'flat trace' or the electronic term 'silent trace' is used to describe variability of <5 BPM. The controlling centre for cardio-acceleration and deceleration is in the medulla area of the brain. Variability is affected by:

- hypoxia – flat trace, sinusoidal patterns (smooth, sinewave pattern of 5–15 BPM recurring 3–5 times per minute lasting more than 10 minutes)
- depressant drugs, e.g. opiates, diazepam – flat trace
- anaemia – sinusoidal patterns
- machinery averaging techniques – display trace with less variability
- neural tube abnormalities affecting control centre, e.g. anencephaly – flat trace
- Doppler technique for fetal heart rate – produces a 'noisy' or irregular trace masking true variability.

A flat trace for less than 20 minutes is non-reassuring or suspicious and is abnormal if the duration is longer than 20 minutes. Note fetal sleep pattern (up to 40 minutes). Interpret by considering all aspects, e.g. the trace of associated deceleration patterns.

Transient changes in heart rate

The fetus is subjected to compression and transient hypoxic stress during uterine contractions. Contractions above 4–6 kPa interrupt placental intervillous blood flow. The healthy fetus tolerates these impositions without many changes in heart rate. With fetal compromise and/or non-physiological uterine contractions, patterns of transient fetal heart rate changes are observed, reflecting the degree of fetal response. It takes 60–90 seconds for reoxygenation of the intervillous blood, hence contraction intervals should not be less than 120 seconds.

Transient acceleration

An increase in heart rate (15 BPM or more and lasting 15 or more seconds) throughout contraction is an early response to sympathetic stimuli (Fig. 10.2) and reflects a fetus in good condition.

Early decelerations

An early deceleration is indicated by a decrease in heart rate (15 BPM or more and lasting 15 seconds or more) with the onset of contractions and a return to baseline rate at the end of the contraction (Fig. 10.3). Vagal stimulation, the oxygen conserving diving reflex and response to hypoxia all contribute to this pattern of heart rate change.

Combined patterns – variable decelerations

Between early and late decelerations are patterns where there is a mixture of accelerations and decelerations, suggesting varying severity of stress intermediate between the pure patterns. These patterns are considered to be associated with umbilical vein compression. Patterns where acceleration precedes deceleration indicate possible

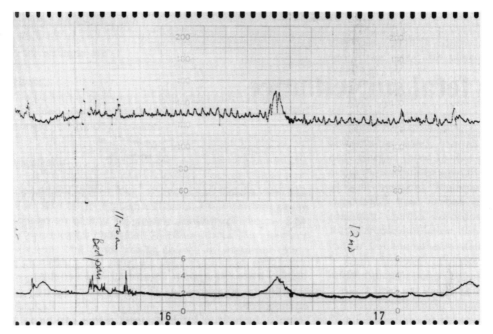

Figure 10.2 Example of transient acceleration in the heart rate.

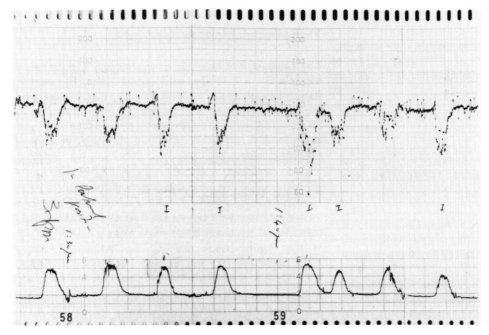

Figure 10.3 Example of a flat trace, early deceleration and combined patterns of acceleration/deceleration in the heart rate.

lesser fetal compromise than decelerations with rebound accelerations. Patterns with slow return to baseline, biphasic deceleration and lots of variability are atypical and suggest abnormality. There is also variable timing of deceleration against uterine contraction.

Late decelerations

Fetal hypoxic insult is suggested by decelerations commencing after mid to end of contraction and nadir is more than 20 seconds after peak of contraction. Decelerations may be shallow or deep. A long lag time or delay before decelerations, a prolonged nadir (more than 3 minutes) or slow return to baseline signifies more severe compromise (Fig. 10.4). Evidence from studies and international consensus advise significance only if the patterns recur and persist.

IMPROVING FETAL HEART RATE RECORDING

Doppler ultrasound techniques (via abdominally-placed transducers) may produce poor quality recordings. Application of a fetal scalp clip (see Box 10.1) gives more satisfactory and more easily interpretable records. These clips may also be applied to the fetal buttocks when the fetus presents by the breech.

Contemporary interpretation of fetal heart rate tracing advises assessment of fetal welfare based on the baseline rate, baseline variability and

---

Box 10.1   Application of scalp clip

- The mother can be in either the dorsal semi-Fowler or the lateral position for application.
- Aseptic precautions are essential.
- Select the appropriate available clip (Fig. 10.5).
- Perform a vaginal examination to determine cervical dilatation, confirm the rupture of membranes and establish presentation of the fetus.
- Direct the clip to a safe area of the scalp or gluteal surface (away from the face, the fontanelle or the fetal perineum).
- Check correct application by examining display of the fetal heart rate on the monitor.
- Anchor the extravaginal part of the clip to the mother's thigh, making sure allowance is made for some slack to accommodate movement (Fig. 10.6).
- Note: do not apply clips if there is a fetal bleeding disorder or if the mother carries the HIV or *Herpes simplex* virus.

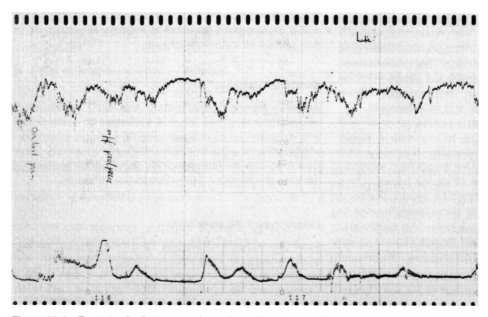

Figure 10.4   Example of a flat trace, tachycardia and late deceleration.

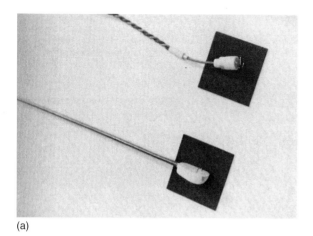

(a)

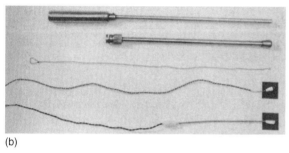

(b)

Figure 10.5   (a) Example of the scalp clips used for direct fetal heart rate monitoring and (b) with applicator.

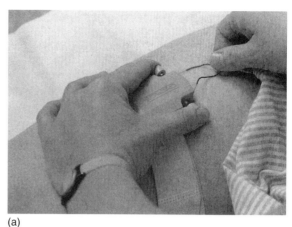

(a)

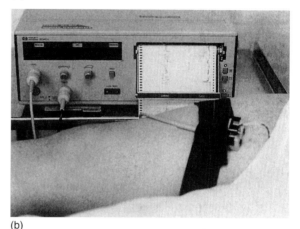

(b)

Figure 10.6   (a) and (b) Anchorage of a clip to thigh.

presence or absence of accelerations and decelerations (early, late and variable).

1. Reassuring trace is one where the baseline rate is between 110 and 160 BPM, variability is 5–25 BPM, with accelerations and no decelerations.

2. Non-reassuring or suspicious trace displays the above described non-reassuring features in rate and variability. Early and variable decelerations are present but no accelerations.

3. An abnormal or pathological trace display a rate below 100 or above 180 BPM, variability is <5 BPM for more than 90 minutes, or there are sinusoidal patterns (over 10 minutes) and the presence of late or atypical variable decelerations.

Requirements for electronic heart rate monitoring

- Ensure compromised or at risk fetuses are offered the benefit of electronic fetal heart rate monitoring.

- Check that the CTG machines are regularly serviced and standardized, for example the running paper speed should be 1 cm per minute.
- All medical staff engaged in the use of electronic FHR monitoring must receive training and regular updating to maintain competency. Training includes drills to respond appropriately when non-reassuring or pathological patterns are detected.
- The FHR trace is a medical record. Events, timing and medical staff involved must be carefully documented on the trace.
- It is a requirement that these fetal heart rate traces are kept for a minimum of 25 years.

Fetal heart rate pattern changes

Labour is associated with progressively stronger and more frequent uterine contractions, hence increasing fetal stress. When fetal compromise is present this increase in neurological and hypoxic stimuli initiates a progression of fetal heart rate pattern changes displaying the range across no response, transient acceleration, early decelerations, variable decelerations and late decelerations. In certain circumstances, such as excessive oxytocic usage or immediately after placement of an epidural block, simple measures such as reduction in oxytocic administration, placing the mother on her side and/or dispense of oxygen with a face-mask for a short time can revert these changes. Many sequences of pattern changes and recovery throughout labour forewarn of the need for a short second stage.

Incomplete progress of patterns

The recognized sequence of fetal heart rate changes from innocuous to non-reassuring and pathological patterns and back again in response to circumstantial situations, such as mother using bedpan or positional postural hypotension, contributes to the acknowledged difficulty in interpretation of fetal heart rate traces.

Palisade patterns

The combination of hypoxia and vagal stimuli at the second stage of labour often produces deep decelerations with usually rapid recovery after each contraction. Deep (less than 100 BPM) heart rate decelerations and tall amplitudes of contraction combine to give the appearance of a fence, hence the term palisade patterns. When these patterns occur, assess cervical dilatation. Since there is a hypoxic component these patterns must not be allowed to continue for too long.

Display of uterine contractions

An external tocometer only indicates the presence of a contraction. The amplitude of the trace displayed on the recording chart is not representative of the intrauterine pressure. Compared with excursions recorded simultaneously from an intrauterine recording system, excursions registered by an external tocometer can precede or follow those derived from an intrauterine system. Classically, early and late decelerations refer to the situation where an intrauterine measuring system is used. Decelerations cannot be timed with accuracy when external tocometers are used because correct placement is often difficult. This statement is particularly important for correct interpretation of fetal heart rate recordings.

Measurements of uterine contractions

Tocometer

An external tocometer (Fig. 10.7) has a button or disc which is depressed when the uterus firms during a contraction (Fig. 10.8). The tocometer is placed at the most convex area of the uterus during contraction to obtain a good display on the recording chart. The amplitude of the contraction displayed is less obvious in overweight mothers. Frequent alteration of the recording site throughout labour is necessary to obtain good displays. External tocometers have the advantage that they can be used when membranes are not ruptured.

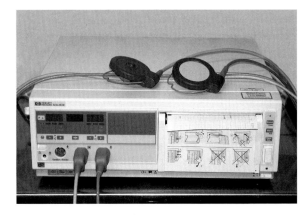

Figure 10.7 Example of an external tocometer.

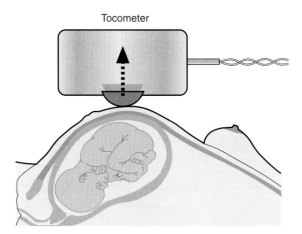

Tocometer

Figure 10.8 The signal is generated by depression of button by mother's abdomen.

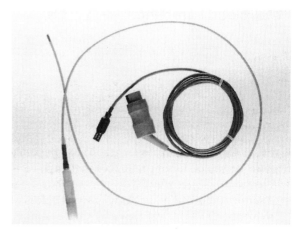

Figure 10.9 Pressure-tipped catheter.

Catheter–transducer system

A saline-filled polythene catheter is placed through the cervix into the amniotic cavity to record the hydrostatic pressure during contractions. This hydrostatic pressure is measured by a transducer with a strain gauge. It requires constant attention (flushing to avoid blockage). There is a risk of infection. When amniotic fluid is reduced towards the end of labour, the amplitude of the displayed excursions becomes less representative of true intrauterine pressure. This system is used to produce the classic descriptions for fetal heart rate recordings. It has been largely superseded by pressure-tipped catheter systems.

Pressure-tipped catheter

A closed system is placed at the tip of a catheter to register increased intrauterine pressure. Increased hydrostatic pressure causes an alteration in the electrical frequency response of the transducer system which is displayed to reflect the intensity of uterine contractions. It is convenient, less affected by alterations between the level of the uterus and the recording transducer, and is more acceptable to the mother and attendant staff (Fig. 10.9). Avoid entrapment of catheter tip. (The tip should be free in the amniotic cavity.)

FETAL ACID-BASE BALANCE

Fetal pH

Fetal hypoxia promotes anaerobic metabolism and the production of lactic acid which accumulates to lower fetal pH (pH = the logarithm of the reciprocal of hydrogen ion concentration, expresses presence or absence of acidaemia). The pH at the onset of labour in a normal fetus is about 7.33 (range 7.20–7.50). There is a slight drop to 7.27 at the time of delivery. This is due to accumulation of lactic acid generated during transient hypoxia associated with contractions. Fetal acidaemia correlates poorly with the Apgar score of the newborn. Acidaemia is evident in 2% of uncomplicated births and most of these babies do not develop cerebral palsy.

The measurement of base excess in fetal capillary blood gives further insight into the acid-base status of the fetus. Base excess in mEq/l or mmol/l is the amount of acid or base needed to titrate the blood sample to a pH of 7.40 at a PCO_2 of 40 mmHg and a temperature of 37°C. Metabolic acidosis means that the available buffer base is used up and a state of base insufficiency or base deficit exists. The prefix minus (–) denotes a negative balance of buffer bases. Normal umbilical artery base excess is in the range of 6.7 mEq/l. In acute anoxia the pH falls by 0.1 units per minute. Negative base excess or base deficit of more than –12 mEq/l suggests the presence of acidaemia.

Fetal blood sampling

The pH of capillary blood from the fetal scalp or the gluteal area should be checked whenever fetal compromise is suspected.

Procedure

- Place the mother in the lithotomy position with 15° lateral tilt or preferably in a left lateral position.
- Aseptic precautions include gowns, gloves, cleansing of the vulval area and sterile drapes.
- Check that the cervical dilatation is 3 cm or more with easy access to fetus.
- Select an amnioscope of the appropriate size and digitally guide it through the cervix onto the fetal skin. Remove the obturator and attach a light source. Alternatively the speculum or an endoscope can be guided through the cervix under direct vision with a fibreoptic light attached.
- Apply the endoscope firmly to the fetal skin to exclude seepage of amniotic fluid.
- Rub the fetal skin with a swab to clean it and use ethyl chloride spray to produce reactive hyperaemia.
- Coat the skin surface with silicone gel so the blood will form a globule. For a hairy surface, part or remove the hair to prevent smudging of the blood trickle.
- Press the prepared skin firmly once or twice with a 2 mm guarded blade (Fig. 10.10) to make an incision.

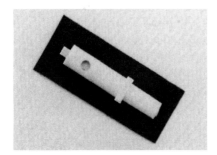

Figure 10.10 Guarded blade to induce capillary ooze.

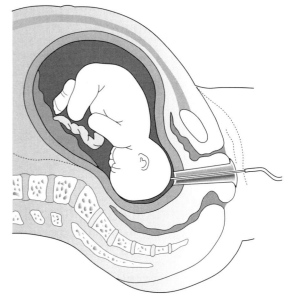

Figure 10.11 Fetal blood sampling.

- Collect the blood into heparinized capillary tubes by gravitation (Fig. 10.11). Suction through a tube is not advised because of potential risk of infection.
- Collect sufficient blood for three consecutive readings. Tubes are sealed after a small segment of iron filing ('flea') is inserted. This filing is moved up and down the tube with a magnet to mix the blood.
- Apply pressure or silicone wax to the incision to secure haemostasis.
- Process samples immediately (Fig. 10.12). Prolonged exposure to air will raise pH.
- In the breech presentation blood from the buttocks is interpreted in the same way as in cephalic presentation.
- Fetal blood sampling is contraindicated when there is maternal infection, e.g. HIV, *Herpes simplex;* presence of fetal bleeding disorders, e.g. haemophilia; or prematurity of less than 34 weeks.

Drill for abnormal fetal heart rate trace

General principles and care paths are as follows:

- Try to determine cause.

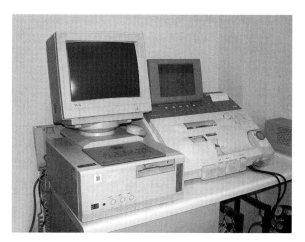

Figure 10.12 Example of blood gas analyser for measuring fetal pH and base excess.

- Check maternal pulse, blood pressure and medication. Is mother in pain, anxious or febrile?
- Turn mother on her side. Select side away from placental bed (normally turn to left side away from inferior vena cava).
- Adjust or switch off intravenous oxytocin. Give tocolytic, e.g. subcutaneous terbutaline 0.25 mg if hypercontractility persists.
- Assess cervical dilatation. Exclude cord prolapse.
- If appropriate give the mother oxygen by using a facemask. Avoid prolonged use of oxygen as it can be harmful to the fetus.
- Expedite delivery if the cervix is fully dilated and there are no contraindications.
- Sample fetal blood if cervix is not fully dilated.
- Assess the total clinical situation. Caesarean section and early delivery can be more appropriate than performing fetal blood sampling, e.g. in deceleration of more than 3 minutes.
- Notify paediatrician/neonatologist.
- Check pH and base excess of cord blood (arterial and venous) at delivery when there is evidence of intrapartum fetal compromise, need for assisted delivery or if baby is delivered in poor condition.

Further points

- Use your common sense. When fetal heart rate changes indicate severe compromise in an at-risk fetus, immediate delivery rather than fetal blood sampling is appropriate. Consider delivery rather than repeat sampling if there is fetal compromise and the fetal pH is borderline (7.21–7.25).
- With complete anoxia pH falls at a rate of 0.1 pH units per minute. The interval between repeat sampling must be flexible and should be guided by close observation of the fetal heart rate.
- Acidaemia is accepted as being present when the fetal pH is less than 7.20. With pH of 7.21–7.25 repeat in 15–30 minutes or consider delivery if non-reassuring fetal heart rate abnormalities persist. Consider base deficit results.
- Maternal lactic acidaemia aggravated by hyperventilation can add to fetal acidosis as there is free transplacental interchange of acid metabolites. The fetal scalp pH is 0.1 pH units below that of the maternal venous blood. A fetal pH of more than 0.2 pH units below that of the maternal venous blood means that fetal acidosis is independent of any maternal influence.
- A fetal scalp caput, uterine contractions and the occasional bubble in the collecting tube should not influence pH readings.

FETAL ACIDAEMIA APGAR SCORES AND NEUROLOGICAL OUTCOME

It is accepted that there is disconcordance between fetal heart rate, fetal acidaemia, subsequent Apgar scores and eventual neurological sequelae. The fetal acid base status should be checked when the fetal heart rate patterns show persistence of a non-reassuring or pathological trace.

When there is disconcordance between the fetal heart rate trace and fetal pH, check acid base status within 30 minutes. In the presence of continuing pathological patterns the fetus should be delivered. Cord blood pH and base deficit status should be checked after delivery.

MECONIUM AND MECONIUM ASPIRATION

- Meconium (Greek word for opium poppy) is present in the fetal gut from 10 weeks gestation. Passage into the amniotic fluid is uncommon before 34 weeks but is detected in 14–30% of pregnancies by 40 weeks (up to 50% at 42 weeks) and reflects gastrointestinal maturity.
- Meconium in amniotic fluid is also more likely if a fetus weighs more than 4000 g and mothers are of African origin (1.5 times more likely compared to mothers of Caucasian origin).
- Parasympathetic activity mediated by the hypothalamus, local peristaltic reflexes and the intestinal hormone motilin all contribute to passage of meconium.
- Infection will produce fetal enteritis which initiates passage of meconium even in the preterm fetus.
- Hypoxia per se does not lead to passage of meconium. In the presence of normal fetal heart rate patterns fetal outcome is similar with or without meconium in the amniotic fluid.
- It is difficult to determine the exact time when meconium is passed.
- Meconium aspiration is defined as presence of meconium below the vocal chords and occurs in 35% of babies when amniotic fluid is meconium stained.
- Most meconium aspiration occurs in utero associated with fetal gasping (response to hypoxaemia) but not irregular deep breathing, which increases with fetal maturity. The fetus inhales 200 ml/kg/24 h of amniotic fluid.
- Meconium aspiration is more likely when meconium concentration is described as thick (usually reflecting the presence of oligohydramnios) and if the pH is <7.20.
- Aspirated meconium damages the fetal lungs by its biochemical properties and furthermore predisposes to infective pneumonitis.
- In the absence of hypoxia aspiration is asymptomatic in 90% of babies or is only associated with mild disease. Meconium aspiration is usually (95%) associated with thick meconium and when severe and compounded by hypoxia predicts a high neonatal death rate (up to 40%).

Management of meconium in amniotic fluid

- Check and record presence of meconium after membrane rupture.
- Fetal blood sampling is not indicated if fetal heart rate is normal.
- The presence of non-reassuring fetal heart rate patterns indicates that risk of fetal acidaemia is increased. Check fetal pH.
- Amnio-infusion cannot prevent passage or inhalation of meconium but only dilutes its concentration. Its value awaits confirmation.
- Pharyngeal aspiration if performed must be gentle to avoid trauma and expedient to prevent further risk of hypoxia.
- When meconium stained amniotic fluid is evident continuous fetal heart rate monitoring is advised. By the same token avoid maternal hypotension, maternal hypoxia, excessive uterine contractions or situations which may precipitate fetal hypoxia.
- Aspirate the oropharynx then the nose as soon as the fetal head is delivered.
- A paediatrician/neonatologist should attend the deliveries.

OTHER CONSIDERATIONS
Severe moulding

Fetal skull bones are not fused, thus permitting a certain amount of movement (separation or overlap) when the fetal head adjusts during its passage through the maternal pelvis. This adjusting or moulding is noticed first at the occipital–parietal sutures. The next suture involved is the parietal–frontal suture and lastly the parietal–parietal suture. Moulding is described as of minor degree when the bones just approximate. Overlapping of bones which can be readily separated digitally is observed with further moulding. Severe moulding is evident when the overlapping bones cannot be separated. Severe moulding is associated with fetal heart rate decelerations, lower pH value and poor Apgar scores hence is considered a signal for fetal compromise. Where there is overlapping, the situation must be reviewed and delivery considered if it is not safe to continue labour.

Fetal movements

Excessive or turbulent fetal movements are sometimes observed during labour and should be viewed with concern as indicative of fetal compromise. Steps should be taken to check the fetal heart rate pattern and if necessary the fetal pH.

REFERENCES

Department of Health 1995 Confidential enquiries into stillbirth and deaths in the UK 1993. HMSO, London

Maternal and Child Health Consortium 2000 Confidential enquiry into stillbirth and deaths in infancy (CESDI) – 7th annual report. HMSO, London

National Institute for Clinical Excellence 2001 Clinical guidelines. The use of electronic fetal monitoring. RCOG, London

FURTHER READING

Alexander G R, Hulsey TC, Robillard PY et al 1994 Determinants of meconium stained amniotic fluid in term pregnancies. Journal of Perinatology 14: 259–263

Baker P N, Kilby M D, Murray H 1992 An assessment of the use of meconium alone as an indication for fetal blood sampling. Obstetrics and Gynecology 80: 792–796

Beard R W, Morris E D, Clayton S G 1967 pH of fetal capillary blood as an indicator of the condition of the fetus. Journal of Obstetrics and Gynecology of the British Commonwealth 74: 812–822

Beard R W, Filshie G M, Knight C A, Roberts G M 1971 The significance of the changes in the continuous fetal heart rate in the first stage of labour. Journal of Obstetrics and Gynecology of the British Commonwealth 78: 865–880

Becker R F, Windle W F, Barth E E, Schulz M D 1940 Fetal swallowing, gastro-intestinal activity and defaecation in utero. Surgery Gynaecology Obstetrics 70: 603–614

Brotanek V, Hendricks C H, Yoshida T 1969 Changes in uterine blood flow during uterine contractions. American Journal of Obstetrics and Gynecology 103: 1108–1116

Cree J E, Meyer J Hailey D M 1973 Diazepam in labour: its metabolism and effect on the clinical condition and thermogenesis of the newborn. British Medical Journal 4: 251–255

Duenholter J H, Pritchard J A 1976 Fetal respiration: quantitative measurements of amniotic fluid inspired near term by human and rhesus fetuses. American Journal of Obstetrics and Gynecology 125: 306–309

Duenholter J H, Pritchard J A 1977 Fetal respiration: a review. American Journal of Obstetrics and Gynecology 129: 326–338

Falciglia H S 1988 Failure to prevent meconium aspiration syndrome. Obstetrics and Gynecology 71: 349–353

Fleischer A, Schulman H, Jagani N et al 1982 The development of fetal acidosis in the presence of an abnormal fetal heart rate tracing. American Journal of Obstetrics and Gynecology 144: 55–60

Gonalez D E, Dios J et al 1998 Neonatal morbidity associated with meconium amniotic fluid. Annals of Espana Paediatricia 48: 54–59

Guyton A C 1991 Behavioural and motivational mechanisms of the brain, the limbic system and the hypothalamus. In: Textbook of physiology, 8th edn. W B Saunders, Philadelphia, p 651–656

Hobbel C J, Hyvarinen M A, Oh W 1972 Abnormal fetal heart rate patterns and fetal acid base balance in low birthweight infants in relation to the respiratory distress syndrome. Obstetrics and Gynecology 39: 83–88

Liu D T Y, Thomas G, Blackwell R J 1975 Progression in response patterns of fetal heart rate throughout labour. British Journal of Obstetrics and Gynaecology 82: 943

Low J A 1997 Intrapartum fetal asphyxia: definition, diagnosis and classification. American Journal of Obstetrics and Gynecology 176: 957–959

Low J A, Cox M J, Karchmar E J et al 1981 The prediction of intrapartum fetal metabolic acidosis by fetal heart rate monitoring. American Journal of Obstetrics and Gynecology 139: 299–335

MacLennan A 2000 A template for defining a causal relationship between acute intrapartum events and cerebral palsy. International Consensus Statement. Australian and New Zealand Journal of Obstetrics and Gynaecology 40: 1322

Mohmoud E L, Benirschke K, Vaucher Y E, Poitras P 1988 Motilin levels in term neonates who have passed meconium prior to birth. Journal of Paediatric Gastroenterology and Nutrition 7: 95–99

Moss D, Holm B A, Spitale P et al 1991 Inhibition of pulmonary surfactant function by meconium. American Journal of Obstetrics and Gynecology 164: 477–481

Naeye R L, Peters E C, Bartholomew M, Landis J R 1989 Origins of cerebral palsy. American Journal of Diseases of Children 143: 1154–1161

Romero R, Hanaoka S, Manzor M et al 1991 Meconium stained amniotic fluid: a risk factor for microbial invasion of the amniotic cavity. American Journal of Obstetrics and Gynecology 164: 859–862

Rossi E M, Philipson E H, Williams T G, Kalhan S C 1989 Meconium aspiration syndrome: intrapartum and neonatal attributes. American Journal of Obstetrics and Gynecology 161: 1106–1110

Schulze M 1925 The significance of the passage of meconium during labour. American Journal of Obstetrics and Gynecology 10: 83–88

Sedaghatian M, Otman L, Hossain M M et al 2001 Risk of meconium staining amniotic fluid in different ethnic groups. Journal of Perinatology 20: 257–261

Steer P J, Eigbe F, Lissauer T J, Beard R W 1989 Inter-relationships among abnormal cardiotocograms in labour, meconium staining of the amniotic fluid, arterial cord blood pH and Apgar scores. Obstetrics and Gynecology 74: 715–721

Stewart K S, Philpott R H 1981 Fetal response to cephalo–pelvic disproportion. British Journal of Obstetrics and Gynaecology 87: 641–649

Sykes G, Molloy P M, Johnson P et al 1982 Do Apgar scores indicate asphyxia? Lancet 1: 494–495

Umstad M P, Permeezel M, Pepperell R J 1994 Intrapartum cardiotocography and the expert witness. Australia and New Zealand Journal of Obstetrics and Gynaecology 34: 20–23

Winkler C L, Hauth J C, Tucker J M et al 1991 Neonatal complications at term as related to the degree of umbilical artery acidaemia. American Journal of Obstetrics and Gynecology 164: 637–641

Yeomans E R, Gilstrap L C, Lebeno K J, Vurris J S 1989 Meconium in the amniotic fluid and fetal acid base status. Obstetrics and Gynecology 73: 175–178

11

Episiotomy and tears

D. Liu

Episiotomy is the term for an incision in the perineum. Not all mothers require an episiotomy for delivery but considerable experience is necessary to determine when it is not needed. This incision is made:

- when a perineal tear is imminent, thus avoiding uncontrolled damage
- to relieve pressure on the soft preterm fetal head
- to expedite delivery when birth is delayed by an unyielding perineum
- to provide adequate room for assisted delivery.

TYPES OF INCISIONS

Medial incision

Medial incisions are made in the anatomical plane and are comfortable. There is less bleeding and they are easy to repair. However, access is limited and the incision carries the risk of extension into the rectum, hence it is only used by someone experienced (Fig. 11.1a).

Mediolateral incision

This incision is safe, easy to perform and thus the most commonly used. The cut must begin at the midpoint of the fourchette and is directed towards the ischial tuberosity into the ischiorectal pad of fat (Fig. 11.1).

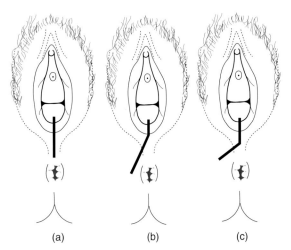

Figure 11.1 (a) Medial incision, (b) mediolateral incision, (c) J-shaped incision.

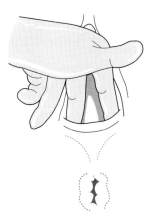

Figure 11.2 Using the fingers the fourchette is drawn away from the presenting part of the fetus before infiltration.

J-shaped incision

This type of incision has the advantage of the medial incision and provides better access than the mediolateral approach. The lateral incision is made tangential to the brown of the anus (Fig. 11.1c). It is excellent for the experienced surgeon.

TECHNIQUE

- An existing epidural can provide adequate anaesthesia; if not, infiltrate with a local anaesthetic. The fingers are placed inside the introitus to protect the presenting parts of the fetus (Figs 11.2 and 11.3).
- The index and middle fingers are placed in the introitus along the direction of the intended cut. The thumb is apposed to stabilize the perineum. A single cut 3 cm long starting from the midpoint of the fourchette is made with scissors.
- In the J-shaped incision, the thumb, middle and index fingers are apposed in the midline of the fourchette. The tip of the thumb is placed 0.5–1 cm above the brown of the anus. A midline incision to the tip of the thumb is made. The thumb and fingers are kept firmly apposed. The scissors are then rotated to align

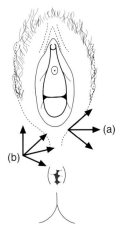

Figure 11.3 Infiltration of local anaesthetic in fan formation starting either at (a) middle of fourchette, or (b) near ischial tuberosity to cover area of incision.

transgentially to the brown perianal area and a further incision is then made (Fig. 11.4).

TIMING

Episiotomy should be performed:

- when tearing of the vagina becomes obvious. This is indicated by a show of fresh blood when the presenting part of the fetus distends the perineum as the mother pushes;
- when the overstretched perineum may be seen to tear;
- electively with a thick unyielding perineum;

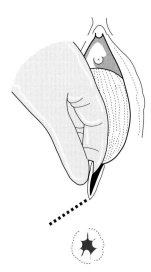

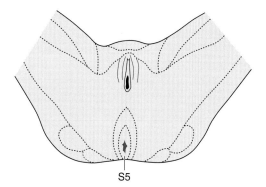

Figure 11.5 Dermatomes of the perineum. Perianal area is supplied by S5.

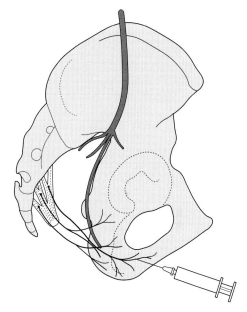

Figure 11.4 Performing a J-shaped episiotomy.

- electively before traction on the forceps or before proceeding to breech delivery (when a breech is on the perineum).

DO

- Place the mother in the lithotomy position.
- Unless in an emergency, ensure there is adequate anaesthesia. Epidural anaesthesia may not be sufficient. Pudendal block anaesthetizes only S2–S4 hence perineal infiltration with additional local anaesthetic is required to cover S5 of the perianal area (Fig. 11.5).
- Remember the total amount of local anaesthetic used should not exceed 200 mg of lignocaine. This is especially important in mothers with an epidural block.
- The pudendal nerve enters the pudendal canal approximately 1 cm below and 1 cm cephalid to the ischial spine when the mother is supine. The pudendal vessels are beside the nerves (Fig. 11.6), therefore aspirate back before infiltration to prevent intravascular injection.
- Perform episiotomy with one or two strokes and not with multiple bites.
- In repeat episiotomies follow the previous properly made incisions.
- If an episiotomy must be made before the perineum is fully stretched by the presenting

Figure 11.6 Pudendal nerve crosses ischial spine medial to the pudendal artery.

part of the fetus, simulate that situation by applying gentle traction on the perineum before making the incision. This will reduce the bulk of tissue incised, hence minimizing bleeding and trauma.

- Tie off or place a clip on any spurting vessels to reduce blood loss. For the same reason repair episiotomies as soon as possible.
- Ensure the apex of the incision is identified before repair. If there is extension into the fornices a general anaesthetic or epidural block

will aid proper exploration of damage and subsequent repair.

- Check the vaginal incision for any gaps in the suturing. Finally examine the rectal aspect of the incision. Any stitch through into the rectum should be cut to prevent infection and fistula formation. Ensure haemostasis is achieved.

DO NOT

- Perform the episiotomy too early because vaginal delivery may not be possible, and blood loss and discomfort are increased when mothers receive both a perineal and an abdominal incision.
- When obstruction to ready delivery is due to a thick or unyielding posterior fourchette (Fig. 11.7). Do not incise beyond this obstruction.
- Do not incise beyond the bony ischial tuberosities. Outlet obstruction due to bony structures is not relieved by an episiotomy. A generous episiotomy is not generous for the mother.
- Do not make an episiotomy before rotation with Kielland's forceps. Vaginal delivery may

not be achieved and rotation can extend the episiotomy.

- Do not leave any vaginal pack behind.
- Do not pull stitches too tight. This only increases discomfort and oedema.

REPAIR OF EPISIOTOMY

- Mothers should be in the lithotomy position. Cleanse the surgical field, drape and maintain aseptic technique. Commence suturing from above the apex and appose the vaginal mucosa continuous with locking stitches placed 1 cm apart and 1 cm from the edge of the wound. Tie off at the vaginal mucocutaneous junction of the fourchette (Figs 11.8a, 11.8b). Ensure anatomical apposition especially at hymenal remnants and mucocutaneous junction.
- This is followed by interrupted sutures placed perpendicular to the skin (Fig. 11.8b). These sutures occlude any dead space and appose subcutaneous tissue, levator ani and perineal muscles. Avoid putting sutures through the rectal mucosa.
- The subcutaneous sutures are placed 1 cm deep and 1 cm apart to close the cutaneous wound. Polyglycolic sutures which produce less tissue reaction are recommended (Figs 11.8c, 11.8d).
- Check the vagina to ensure no gaps are present in the suture line and haemostasis is achieved. Perform a rectal examination to exclude any stitch which may have come through the rectal mucosa and presence of a haematoma. Any rectal stitch must be cut. A haematoma must be evacuated.

RESUTURING EPISIOTOMIES

Breakdown of an episiotomy often follows infection of a haematoma. The following procedures should be adopted:

- Take swabs from the infected wound and vagina for bacterial culture.
- Epidural or general anaesthesia facilitates proper repair.
- The old episiotomy must be opened up in total, the haematoma if present is evacuated, the

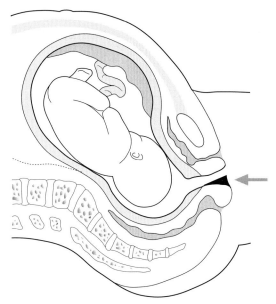

Figure 11.7 Obstruction caused by unyielding posterior fourchette (shaded) area.

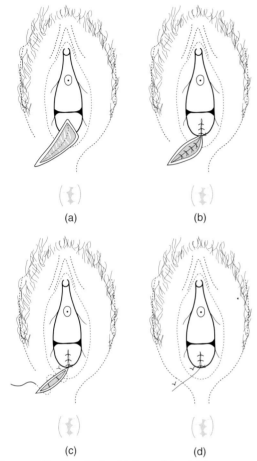

Figure 11.8 Repair of episiotomy: (a) episiotomy, (b) continuous locking vaginal stitches and interrupted sutures, (c) subcutaneous sutures, (d) repair complete. Step (c) can be replaced by interrupted sutures.

wound edges freshened and the repair effected by interrupted sutures to allow drainage.

- Superficial dehiscence of the wound edges need not be resutured. Keeping the wound clean by regular bathing with salt and water will promote rapid healing by secondary intention.

TEARS IN THE PERINEUM

Eighty-five per cent of vaginal deliveries are associated with some perineal trauma. These are graded into:

- first degree – superficial lacerations, underlying muscles not damaged

- second degree – lacerations involving tearing of perineal muscles
- third degree – damage involving partial or complete disruption of external anal sphincter
- fourth degree – there is complete disruption of external and internal sphincter and rectal mucosa.

Tearing is associated with:

- primiparous delivery
- prolonged second stage of labour
- narrow subpubic arch
- poorly flexed head and occipital posterior position
- precipitate labour
- big baby (more than 4000 g)
- shoulder dystocia
- assisted vaginal delivery (e.g. forceps – but much less with Ventouse extractions).

Superficial grazes and tears, if they are not bleeding, can be left. Second degree tears are repaired as for episiotomies. Skin edges, because they are ragged, may need interrupted rather than subcutaneous sutures.

Vaginal delivery with mediolateral episiotomy is associated with possible 4% (range 0.6–9.0%) third and fourth degree tears. Severe tears are more common in the nullipara (4%), birthweight over 4 kg (2%), occipitoposterior position (3%), long second stage (4%) and forceps delivery (7%).

Repair of a third degree tear requires:

- Epidural or general anaesthesia (allow anal sphincter to relax and facilitate adequate repair).
- Continuous suture to repair the rectal mucosa. Commence above the apex of the tear; the mucosa is everted into the rectum. Tie off at the mucocutaneous junction (Fig. 11.9a). Use monofilament suture if available.
- The vaginal mucosa is repaired as for an episiotomy (Fig. 11.9b).
- The severed ends of the rectal sphincter, which usually retract, are identified and apposed by interrupted sutures (Fig. 11.9c). End to end repair of the sphincter results in poor subsequent function when the ends

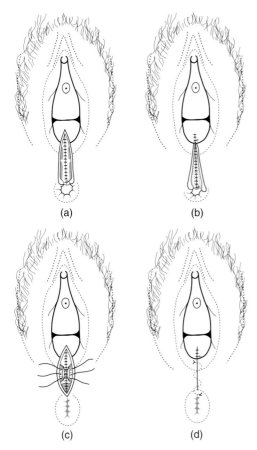

(a)　　　　　　(b)

(c)　　　　　　(d)

Figure 11.9 Repair of third degree tear. Repair of:
(a) rectal mucosa, (b) vaginal mucosa, (c) rectal sphincter,
(d) subcuticular sutures.

retract. Overlapping the ends of the sphincter provides more perineal bulk and better function. The anus should accommodate a finger after the sphincter muscles are approximated. The skin is apposed by subcutaneous and interrupted sutures (Fig. 11.9d). Ensure that the vaginal introitus accepts two fingers at the end of the repair.

- Avoid constipation. A low-fibre diet and faecal softeners are advised, e.g. Lactulose and Fybogel for 10 days. Do not use oil-based aperients. They inhibit healing of wound edges and encourage recto-vaginal fistula formation.

- Prophylactic antibiotics reduce infection and wound dehiscence. Use metronidazole and broad spectrum antibiotics.
- Prescribe adequate postoperative analgesia.
- Advise elective caesarean section for subsequent births since further vaginal delivery increases risk of anal incontinence.

Consequence for mothers of perineal trauma

- In 10% of mothers pain and discomfort will last 3–18 months after delivery.
- 20% will experience superficial dyspareunia for some 3 months.
- 3–10% report faecal incontinence (30% flatus incontinence).
- 20% experience urinary incontinence.
- Occult anal sphincter damage occurs in 36% after vaginal delivery and is evident in 70% (range 54–88%) despite repair of third and fourth degree tears.
- Review mothers with severe tears 6 months or a year after delivery.

Box 11.1 gives further information on third degree tears.

Box 11.1　Third degree tears: faecal incontinence

- Some 13% of mothers experience a degree of incontinence, usually flatus or rectal urgency, after vaginal delivery.
- Faecal incontinence is due to nerve, and external and internal anal sphincter injury. Both nerve and muscle are damaged when injury is severe.
- Mediolateral episiotomy need not prevent third degree tears. Two-thirds of third degree tears occur in mothers with an episiotomy.
- Poor repair will result in subsequent sphincter defect with 50% of mothers having a degree of incontinence (flatus, faecal).
- Some 10% of mothers may experience wound disruption necessitating further surgery.
- All mothers with third degree tears should be reviewed three months after surgery.

FURTHER READING

Bek K M, Laurberg S 1992 Risk of anal incontinence from subsequent vaginal delivery after a complete obstetric and sphincter tear. British Journal of Obstetrics and Gynaecology 99: 724–726

Browning G G, Motson R W 1983 Results of Parks operation for faecal incontinence after anal sphincter injury. British Medical Journal of Clinical Research Education 286: 1873–1875

Royal College of Obstetricians and Gynaecologists 2001 Guideline number 29, 2001. RCOG, London

Sultan A H, Kamm M A, Hudson C N et al 1993 Anal sphincter disruption during vaginal delivery. New England Journal of Medicine 329: 1905–1911

Sultan A H, Kamm M A, Hudson C N, Bartram C I 1994 Third degree obstetric anal sphincter tears and risk factors and outcome of primary repair. British Medical Journal 308: 887–891

Venkatesh K S, Ramanujam P S, Larson D M, Haywood M A 1989 Anorectal complications of vaginal delivery. Diseases of the colon and rectum 32: 1039–1416

Wood J, Amos L, Rieger N 1998 Third degree anal sphincter tears: risk factors and outcomes. Australian and New Zealand Journal of Obstetrics and Gynaecology 38: 414–417

12

The newborn

D. A. Curnock

Next to the risks encountered during labour, the transition from intrauterine to independent extrauterine existence is the second most critical period of the neonate's life. Mismanagement or failure to anticipate difficulties results in unncessary damage to or death of the newborn. At every delivery a person should be present who has been trained in neonatal resuscitation. In addition, a paediatrician or a nurse practitioner with advanced resuscitation skills should be called to attend the delivery when:

- there is poor fetal growth and/or any obstetric complication, including multiple births
- the delivery is preterm
- there is intrapartum fetal distress
- assisted or operative delivery is contemplated
- meconium is present
- there is intrapartum pyrexia
- depressant drugs have been given within three hours of delivery
- there is known serious fetal abnormality.

Aftercare is most effective if:

- all labour ward personnel understand neonatal physiology and are familiar with resuscitative procedures;
- the neonatal condition is assessed accurately and the correct resuscitation measures are promptly undertaken. There is no place for deliberation or a 'wait and see' policy when a baby fails to establish regular respiration;
- well-drilled teamwork is ensured;
- equipment for resuscitation is well maintained.

PHYSIOLOGICAL CONSIDERATIONS

Acid base

Before labour the normal fetus has a pH around 7.3, PCO_2 about 35 mmHg and PO_2 between 35 and 40 mmHg. At the end of labour repeated episodes of hypoxia associated with uterine contractions result in the normal neonate having a pH of 7.22–7.26, PCO_2 of 50 mmHg, PO_2 of 20 mmHg and a base excess of –5 to –8. This change equates with subjecting a normal fetus to 2 minutes of total anoxia. After 8–10 minutes of total anoxia, permanent brain damage would result.

Cardiovascular system

The fetal lungs *in utero* receive only 10% of the fetal right ventricular output. At birth the infant's first breath expands the lungs and reduces pulmonary vascular resistance, thus allowing increased pulmonary flow. At the same time systemic vascular resistance rises when the umbilical cord is clamped. These changes and rising PO_2 result in closure of the shunts, foramen ovale and ductus arteriosus, to establish the pulmonary and systemic circulation. Hypoxia, acidosis and pulmonary atelectasis increase pulmonary vascular resistance and hence prevent closure of the shunts, thus limiting oxygenation of the blood. Prompt resuscitation will:

- encourage expansion of the lungs
- allow ventilation to reduce PCO_2 and increase PO_2
- reduce acidosis.

Breathing is stimulated by exposure to the extrauterine environment and by the increasing fetal plasma carbon dioxide (PCO_2). Air is drawn in during the first breath. However, this air is expelled again through a partly closed glottis to effect the cry we hear from a healthy baby. During the first few minutes, breathing may be irregular or even intermittent but this is followed by more regular breathing at 40–60 breaths a minute. Regular breathing lowers PCO_2 and raises PO_2.

Normal acid-base status is only achieved at the end of 1 or 2 hours. Any complication which depresses the neonate prolongs this recovery period.

Delivery of the fetal nose and mouth

- Once the nose and mouth are delivered, ensure and maintain a clear airway. First suck out the mouth and oropharynx and then the nose.
- Do not apply suction to the nose before the mouth and oropharynx are cleared. Stimulation of the nose will cause the neonate to gasp and inhale the contents in the oropharynx.
- Do not pass the sucker too far into the mouth. Stimulation of the hypopharynx can cause laryngospasm and bradycardia.

Lung liquid

In utero the fetus secretes fluid continuously from its lungs. Compression of the thorax during labour helps to expel this lung fluid. It is thought that raised fetal plasma adrenaline following the stress of labour is important in switching off the mechanism for lung fluid production and thus preparing the fetus for extrauterine existence. The residual lung liquid at birth is usually rapidly absorbed into the capillaries or lymphatics. Infants delivered electively by caesarean section have less opportunity for removing this lung fluid and therefore may develop some respiratory distress (transient tachypnoea) due to retention of lung liquid. Spontaneous resolution is expected and, whilst an increased oxygen concentration may be needed for a time, artificial ventilation is seldom necessary.

Body temperature

The neonate's large surface area to body volume ratio, especially if preterm or of low birthweight, allows rapid cooling. A rapid drop in body temperature increases the need for oxygenation and exacerbates metabolic acidosis. Maintenance of body temperature is therefore particularly important in depressed infants. Failure to maintain adequate body temperature in preterm neonates is a major contributory factor to mortality due to respiratory distress syndrome. All neonates should be dried quickly, wrapped in prewarmed blankets and placed in a warm environment. Most resuscitation trolleys now incorporate an overhead radiant heater which must be switched on well in advance (Fig. 12.1).

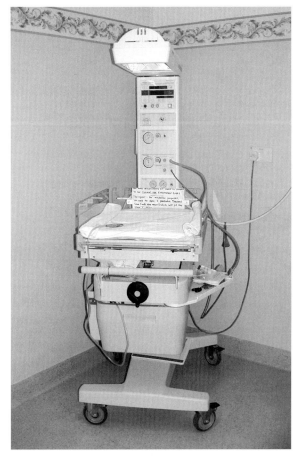

Figure 12.1   Example of resuscitation trolley.

ASSESSMENT OF THE NEWBORN

A system which defines the clinical status of the neonate is important for evaluating the outcome of labour and for documenting the response to resuscitation. The Apgar score, which examines five physical criteria, is the most widely used method (Table 12.1). In pigmented mothers, mucosal colour gives a better guide than skin colour. Each criterion is scored from 0–2 to describe the spectrum from poor to good. The maximum score is 10 points. The baby is examined at 1 minute and again at 5 minutes after birth, scores being allocated at these two intervals. The Apgar score can be repeated again at regular intervals in order to document the response to resuscitation and because later neurodevelopmental disorders increase significantly when scores remain less than 4 for more than 15 minutes.

In order to decide on the baby's need for resuscitation, three of the Apgar score signs are of prime importance – breathing, colour and heart rate. Having assessed the baby it should be assigned to one of four groups, and the appropriate management followed (Table 12.2). Boxes 12.1, 12.2 and 12.3 describe resuscitation procedures and illustrate the use of bag and mask ventilation (Fig. 12.2).

All neonates must be closely observed during the first hour of life. After an initial appearance of wellbeing, the neonate's condition may deteriorate when the stimulus of birth fails to overcome the depressive effects of drugs or central nervous system damage.

In addition to the Apgar score, the biochemical indices of pH and base excess from combined venous and arterial cord blood can provide

Table 12.1   The Apgar score

Physical	Score value		
	0	1	2
Heart rate	Absent	Below 100/min	Over 100/min
Respiratory effort	Absent	Slow, irregular gasping	Good, crying
Muscle tone	Limp/flaccid	Some flexion	Normal with movement
Response to stimulation	No response	Facial grimace	Good response with cry
Colour of trunk	White	Blue	Pink

Table 12.2

Group	Condition at birth	Management
1	Breathing/crying Pink Heart rate >100	Deliver the baby directly onto the mother's abdomen, and dry with a towel. This enhances bonding and maintains temperature by direct skin to skin contact.
2	Apnoeic/gasping Blue Heart rate >100	Stimulate the baby by rubbing the back with a towel or gently tapping the feet. Open and clear the airway by performing gentle oral, followed by nasal suction. Give facial oxygen. If no response is shown by 1 minute of age, i.e. the heart rate is falling or the baby remains blue, then bag and mask ventilation should be commenced. If there is no improvement by 2 minutes of age, i.e. the heart rate has not increased, consider intubating the baby.
3	Apnoeic Blue/pale Heart rate <100	Bag and mask ventilation should be commenced immediately (see Box 12.1). If there is no response within 2 minutes, then intubate the baby.
4	Apnoeic White Heart rate <60	Full cardiopulmonary resuscitation is required. Intubate immediately (see Box 12.2) and commence intermittent positive pressure ventilation (IPPV). If no one experienced at intubation is immediately available, or it is technically difficult, then bag and mask ventilation should be given until help arrives. After 30 seconds reassess heart rate by auscultation. If heart rate is <60 commence external cardiac massage (ECM) (see Box 12.3). N.B. The commonest reason for failure of the heart rate to improve is ineffective lung inflation. Check this is correct before commencing ECM. If there is no response to IPPV and ECM, an umbilical venous catheter should be inserted and adrenaline and sodium bicarbonate given (see Box 12.3).

useful information about the duration of stress suffered and will help guide neonatal resuscitation. Mean cord pH in babies with normal Apgar scores is 7.3. Babies with birth asphyxia usually have cord pH <7.0 but the majority who develop hypoxic ischaemic encephalopathy have pH <6.8.

SPECIAL SITUATIONS

Meconium in the amniotic fluid

- Clear the airways immediately the head is delivered.
- Place the baby on the resuscitation trolley and visualize glottis with laryngoscope. If meconium is present around glottis, intubate immediately and apply direct suction to the tube.
- Maintain suction as the tube is withdrawn. A core of meconium will accompany the tube. Repeat this procedure until the tube comes out clear of meconium. An experienced operator can achieve three or four intubations within the first minute.

- Ventilate with oxygen only when the tube is clear.
- If gasping has occurred and meconium is aspirated, intubate and lavage by instilling 1 ml normal saline down the endotracheal tube, hand ventilate two or three times then suck out. Repeat once or twice.
- If no meconium is seen around the glottis, clear the airways and observe.

Low birthweight infants

Whether due to prematurity or poor intrauterine growth, these infants are susceptible to rapid heat loss and require expert resuscitation.

Hypovolaemic shock (*asphyxia pallida*)

This follows bleeding from the feto–placental vessels (abruptio placentae, placental shunting in twins, intrapartum bleeding and fetal trauma). A poor Apgar score, low circulatory blood volume

Box 12.1 Bag and mask ventilation (Reproduced from RCPCH and RCOG 1997, with permission)

- Airway-opening techniques.
  The head should be tilted back gently to a neutral position and the chin lifted forward taking care not to compress the floor of the mouth.
  A folded towel placed under the neck and shoulders may help to maintain the neutral position.
  Use a 10 FG (black) suction catheter for a term baby or 8 FG (blue) catheter for a preterm baby to gently clear the mouth and pharynx.
- Use a soft silicon mask which is big enough to cover the face from the bridge of the nose to below the mouth. A good seal must be obtained around the infant's face (Fig. 12.2).
- Use a bag with 500 ml capacity and a blow-off valve set at approximately 45 cm H_2O and an oxygen flow rate of 5 l/min.
- The first 5 breaths should be given slowly to establish a functional residual capacity, compressing the bag with the fingers for 1–2 seconds.
- Following the first 5 breaths, ventilation should occur at a rate of 30–40 breaths per minute.
- Observe the chest wall for equal movement and auscultate both lung fields and the stomach to confirm equal bilateral air entry to the lungs. If there is poor inflation check that the airway is not obstructed. Reposition the head, making sure the neck is not over-extended. If necessary perform oral suction.

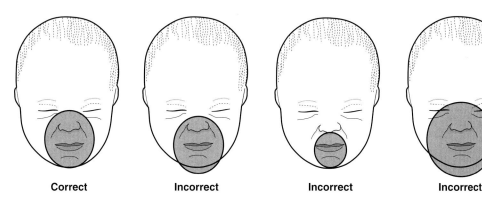

Correct	**Incorrect**	**Incorrect**	**Incorrect**

Figure 12.2 Ensure the correct size and position of the mask.

Box 12.2 Endotracheal intubation and IPPV

- Position baby on resuscitation platform and use airway-opening techniques and suction as for bag and mask ventilation.
- Equipment: a 3 mm endotracheal (ET) tube should be used for a baby ≥32 weeks gestation, and a 2.5 mm ET tube for a baby <32 weeks gestation, with a straight-bladed laryngoscope and a pressure manometer.
  Set the oxygen flow to 5 l/min via a bag and valve or 3–5 l/min via a 'Y' piece.
- Pre-oxygenate the baby using mask ventilation.
- Hold the laryngoscope in the left hand and insert it into the right side of the baby's mouth so that the tip of the blade lies in the oesophagus.
- Use the laryngoscope blade to sweep the tongue across the midline to the left.
- Gently lift the laryngoscope forwards and upwards, withdrawing it very slightly from the oesophagus until the larynx and vocal cords come into view.
- Applying cricoid pressure either by an assistant or by using the little finger of the left hand may be helpful.
- Hold the ET tube with the right hand and gently insert it into the right side of the baby's mouth so that it does not obscure the view of the vocal cords.
- Advance the tip of the ET tube through the cords for 1–2 cm. The approximate length of the ET tube at the lips for infants of 1, 2, and 3 kg respectively is 6.5, 7.5 and 9.0 cm.
- Remove the laryngoscope, and attach the ET tube to the bag and mask or to the 'Y' piece and pressure manometer.
- The first 5 breaths should be held for 2 seconds to establish the functional residual capacity.
- Then ventilate the baby at a rate of 30 breaths per minute.
- Observe chest movement and auscultate over both axillae and over the stomach to assess the correct position of the tube.
- Fix the ET tube, and when the baby is stable check the tube position with a chest X-ray.

N.B. *Never* attach a baby's ET tube to the oxygen supply without a pressure limiting device within the circuit.

Box 12.3 Cardiac arrest

- External cardiac massage (ECM) must be started if there is no heart beat, or the heart rate is <60/min
- The baby will already be receiving IPPV via an endotracheal tube or, if this is not possible, by bag and mask
- There are two techniques
  — the chest is encircled with both hands so that the fingers lie behind the baby and the thumbs are opposed over the sternum
  — two fingers of the same hand are used to compress the sternum
- The thumbs or fingers should be positioned over the middle third of the sternum, 1 cm below the inter-nipple line. The sternum should be compressed to a depth of 1.5–2 cm
- The compressions should be at a rate of 120/min and a ratio of 3 ECM to 1 ventilation
- ECM should continue until the heart rate is >80 beats per minute and increasing
- If there is no response to IPPV and ECM, insert an umbilical venous catheter (UVC)
- Obtain a baseline blood gas, blood sugar, and haemoglobin sample
- Give the following drugs via the UVC:
  — adrenaline 10 micrograms/kg (i.e. 0.1 ml/kg of 1 in 10 000) followed by a 0.5–1.0 ml normal saline flush
  Continue IPPV and ECM. If there is no response, then after 3 minutes give:
  — Sodium bicarbonate (4.2%) 1 mmol/kg (i.e. 2 ml/kg) followed by a saline flush, *and* adrenaline 100 micrograms/kg (i.e. 1 ml/kg of 1 in 10 000) followed by a saline flush
  Further doses of adrenaline 100 micrograms/kg may be given every 3–5 minutes if there is no response
  — 10% glucose. During prolonged resuscitation, test for hypoglycaemia (BM stix <2.1), and if it is present give 10% glucose 5 ml/kg followed by a saline flush.

N.B. All drugs should be checked before giving, and a record of drug administration kept. If there is no response to resuscitation by 20 minutes, then resuscitation should be discontinued, the decision being made by the registrar or consultant.

---

and metabolic acidosis are characteristic. Proceed as follows:

- Resuscitate as for an infant with a poor Apgar score in Group 4 (see Table 12.2).
- Expand the blood volume; uncross-matched O negative whole blood is given. 5–10 ml/kg body weight can be given over 2–3 minutes (normal neonatal blood volume is 70–90 ml/kg).

Shock produces vascular constriction. Following recovery with ventilation or replacement of blood volume, peripheral vessels will dilate and this can cause secondary hypotension and shock. The recovery phase, therefore, must be carefully monitored as relapse after initial recovery may indicate the need for additional replacement.

Drug depression

Drugs used in obstetrics for sedation or analgesia, such as those listed below, will cross the placenta and affect the fetus, causing respiratory depression, poor thermal regulation and depressed reflexes:

- Opiates (pethidine, Omnopon) cause depression if administered to the mother within 3 hours before birth.

  Antidote – naloxone (Narcan) is a specific narcotic antagonist, given intramuscularly or intravenously. There is a wide safety margin and few side effects.

  Dose 5–10 micrograms/kg – most infants can accept 20 micrograms (1 ml Narcan). If there is no response in 1–2 minutes, the depression is not due to narcotics. Naloxone is effective for 1–2 hours. This is shorter than the action of the narcotics, therefore infants must be observed closely for a relapse when further doses of naloxone are required.

- Diazepam (Valium), if more than 30 mg given to the mother in 24 hours, can produce apnoeic spells, carbon dioxide retention and a floppy infant at birth. Keep the baby under close observation, give warmth and support for 24–48 hours. Phenothiazines may produce similar effects in the newborn.

- Chlormethiazole (Heminevrin) for sedation of pre-eclampsia/eclampsia can produce a sleepy baby. There is no specific antidote. Observe, support and keep the baby warm.

- Magnesium sulphate, prescribed for pre-eclampsia, can cause neonatal depression. Antidote – calcium gluconate 100 mg intravenously is effective (30 mg/kg slowly).

- Local anaesthetic. Regional anaesthetic agents administered to the mother can reach the fetus in 30 minutes or less and cause hypotonia and depress myocardial activity. The half-life of these agents in the fetus varies from 3–9 hours. There is no antidote. Observe the baby closely. Gaseous anaesthetic agents can contribute to neonatal depression but these agents are cleared rapidly and therefore present less of a problem.

EMERGENCIES DUE TO CONGENITAL ABNORMALITIES

Certain abnormalities will limit the neonate's ability to establish respiration. Some have a subtle, gradual presentation while others are acute life-threatening conditions.

Choanal atresia

A bony or membranous septum is present across one or both posterior nasal air passages, obstructing breathing.

Presentation

The baby presents with respiratory distress from birth. Neonates are obligatory nose breathers and cannot breathe satisfactorily through the mouth. A catheter cannot pass up through the nostril.

Treatment

Intubate and ensure the baby is comfortable. Replace the endotracheal tube with an oral airway. Resolve the obstruction surgically as a planned procedure.

Upper airway obstruction at vocal cord level

Presentation

The baby presents with respiratory distress and stridor.

Treatment

Ventilation and intubation may not be possible. Tracheostomy or, in less experienced hands, insertion of a wide bore needle into the trachea below the level of the obstruction can allow ventilation until expert help arrives.

Diaphragmatic hernia

There is an incidence of 1 in 4000 live births. Usually the posterolateral part of the diaphragm fails to develop and almost always on the left side.

Presentation

The baby presents with cyanosis, severe respiratory distress, a scaphoid abdomen, poor breath sounds and the heart sound displaced to the right side of the chest. Often diagnosed before birth by routine scanning.

Treatment

Intubate, ventilate and await surgery.

Tracheo-oesophageal fistula (TOF)

This is an additional problem in 90% of babies with oesophageal atresia. Fifty per cent of these babies have congenital heart disease and imperforate anus. The upper oesophageal pouch is usually blind. The distal oesophagus opens into the trachea above its bifurcation (Fig. 12.3).

Presentation

Polyhydramnios is present during pregnancy. At birth we have a mucusy or 'bubbly' baby with

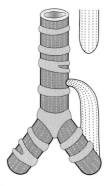

Figure 12.3 Tracheo-oesophageal fistula.

gaseous abdominal distension. Diagnose before first feed to avoid aspiration pneumonia.

Treatment

Pass a wide bore tube (FG 10 or 12), preferably double lumen with radio-opaque line, called a Replogle tube. Aspirate the contents from the upper pouch and X-ray to confirm the level of the blind end. Apply continuous suction on the tube and nurse the baby tilted head up to reduce reflux of gastric acid through fistula until surgery is arranged.

Pulmonary haemorrhage

Bleeding into the alveoli can follow intrapartum pneumonia, severe rhesus disease, intracranial haemorrhage, congenital heart disease and growth retardation with severe intrapartum hypoxia.

Presentation

The infant presents with severe respiratory distress with fresh blood in the trachea. There may be evidence of disseminated intravascular coagulation.

Treatment

Intubate, ventilate using positive end expiratory pressure (PEEP), transfuse with whole blood and isolate cause.

Pneumothorax

This may present spontaneously at birth or occur in association with meconium aspiration or respiratory distress, especially if resuscitation has been over-vigorous.

Prevention

The main danger is tension pneumothorax which rapidly causes respiratory distress and cyanosis. Reduced breath sounds on affected side and cardiac shift suggest pneumothorax but do not indicate the presence or absence of tension. Transillumination with a light source is helpful. Confirm with a chest X-ray if there is no urgency.

Treatment

Aspirate with needle to reduce tension. This must be followed by a chest drain and an underwater seal.

BIRTH TRAUMA (Table 12.3)

Good obstetric practice and better judgement for the mode of delivery have reduced the incidence of birth trauma. It is important to appreciate that sometimes birth trauma can follow an easy spontaneous delivery.

Trauma is most likely in:

- prolonged labour
- trials of labour
- preterm delivery
- operative delivery, and this includes caesarean section.

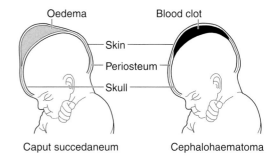

Figure 12.4

Table 12.3

Types of trauma	Description	Causes	Treatment
Minor superficial injuries	Bruises, abrasions, petechiae, subconjunctival haemorrhages, compression marks	Normal delivery, forceps, caesarean sections	Observe baby, reassure mother
Caput succedaneum (substitute head) See also Fig. 12.4	Oedematous swelling over the vertex or occiput	Scalp lymphatics and venous stasis producing a serous collection separating aponeurosis and periosteum. Associated with labour. Degree reflects length and difficulty of labour	Observe spontaneous resolution within 24 hours
Cephalohaematoma See also Fig. 12.4	Well defined swelling over the parietal bone	Collection of blood beneath the periosteum usually of the parietal bone and is limited by the suture lines. Associated with normal delivery, forceps, ventouse extraction, fracture of skull bones	Observe, may increase in size. Resolves in 2–3 weeks. Can contribute to jaundice
Skull fractures	Linear hairline fracture or depressed fractures	Spontaneous deliveries, following trials of labour, assisted deliveries such as forceps or caesarean sections	No treatment unless there is cerebral bleeding, focal neurological irritation or paresis is observed
Subdural haemorrhage	Bulging fontanelle, cerebral irritation, retinal haemorrhage and low Apgar score	Excessive moulding, preterm delivery, difficult forceps, difficult rotation, breech extraction, ruptured veins in the subdural space	Subdural taps. Confirm diagnosis and relieve intracranial pressure
Intracranial haemorrhage	Shocked or stillborn with tear or tears in the tentorium cerebelli identified at post mortem	Spontaneous rapid delivery or follows difficult labour, preterm delivery, breech extraction or assisted delivery	Condition tends to be fatal. If the infant survives lumbar puncture can confirm and ultrasound can be used to localize and determine the extent of bleeding to provide an idea of prognosis
Hypoxic ischaemic encephalopathy	Low Apgar score followed by irritability and high pitched cry. A full fontanelle and tonic convulsions	All events which contribute to fetal hypoxia	Observe, sedate if irritable. Resolution of the condition may be complete or result in various degrees of handicap
Facial palsy	Paralysis of facial muscles, inability to close eye on affected side	Usually follows forceps delivery where the facial nerve is compressed just behind the stylomastoid foramen	Spontaneous recovery within a few days. Apply facial massage to maintain tone. Protect cornea of affected eye
Sternomastoid tumour	Haematoma of the sternomastoid	Rotational delivery, large babies with shoulder problems, breech deliveries after Lovsett manoeuvre	Check the neck of all difficult deliveries. If the condition is missed torticollis may result. Physiotherapy and muscle stretching 3–4 times daily is helpful
Brachial plexus palsy	(a) Erb–Duchenne cervical 5, 6 nerve sheath is torn and nerves compressed by bleeding. Arm on affected side is limp with pronation of forearm and flexion at the wrist (b) Klumpke's cervical 7 and 8 nerve damage. Produces a wrist drop and paralysis of hand	Stretch injury following difficult delivery of the shoulders or difficult Lovsett manoeuvre	Support arm in position of relaxation. Arm is flexed and abducted for Erbs variety of damage. Physiotherapy 3–4 times daily.

Table 12.3 (*Continued*)

Types of trauma	Description	Causes	Treatment
Fractures	Greenstick fractures of limbs or clavicle. Pseudoparalysis or reluctant to move a limb should alert	Mainly with breech delivery or shoulder dystocia. Occasionally may follow normal delivery	Confirm by radiology. Splint to rest affected arm
Visceral damage	Large liver and spleen may be damaged	Breech delivery when the hands are placed too high for the Lovsett manoeuvre particularly in a small or preterm fetus. May also follow vigorous resuscitation	Deteriorating neonatal condition and suspicion of acute abdomen. Necessitates laparotomy

FURTHER READING

Nebon K B, Ellenberg J H 1981 Apgar scores as predictors of chronic neurologic disability. Pediatric 68: 36–44

Richmond S (ed) 1996 Principles of resuscitation at birth, 5th edn. Northern Neonatal Network, Sunderland

RCPCH and RCOG (Royal College of Paediatrics and Child Health and Royal College of Obstetricians and Gynaecologists) 1997 Resuscitation of babies at birth. Report of a joint working party. British Medical Journal Publishing Group, London

13

Preterm labour and preterm premature rupture of membranes

D. Liu, R. Lamont

PRETERM LABOUR

The World Health Organization (ICD10 1992) defined preterm birth as delivery before 37 weeks of pregnancy. Based on this definition 6–10% of births are preterm but around 50% of deliveries are more than 35 weeks gestation with near 100% survival expected of babies born after 32 weeks of pregnancy. Intact survival exceeds 50% after 27 weeks and improves as gestation increases towards 32 weeks. In this group (27–32 week fetus) every effort must be made to enhance survival and optimize quality of life.

The International Classification of Diseases uses 22 completed weeks as the beginning of the perinatal period when birthweight corresponds to 500 g. In practice the lower limit of fetal viability is influenced by available care and varies between 23 and 25 weeks of pregnancy. Delivery at these extreme preterm periods of gestation, 23 weeks to 26 weeks and 6 days, account for the majority of neonatal deaths and subsequent handicaps (75–90% deaths and 50% neurological disabilities, e.g. cerebral palsy).

General statements

When preterm labour presents the following considerations are important:

- Detailed pathophysiology of preterm labour is unknown hence the dilemma for effective therapy. Attempts to improve outcome for this obstetric complication (currently some 13 000 000 preterm deliveries world wide) include efforts to predict or prevent its

Table 13.1 Preterm labour: proposed guidelines for management

Cervical status	Cervical dilatation (cm)	Uterine contraction	Suggested management
Effaced	>3	Nil	Cerclage
Not effaced	≤3	Two in 10 minutes lasting more than 40 seconds for 1 hour	Treat if present for more than 2 hours
Effaced	4–5	As above	Urgent therapy with loading dose regimen
Effaced	≥6	Established labour	Preparation for delivery

occurrence by risk scores, sonographic cervical assessment, uterine activity monitoring or tests for fibronectin presence in cervico-vaginal secretions. Correct diagnosis of labour onset is important (Table 13.1).

- Obstetric associations include congenital fetal abnormality, preterm membrane rupture (30–40%), placental separation, intrauterine infection (10–15%) and fetal death. Perform ultrasound scan to exclude contraindications for therapy.
- Only infection and spontaneous onset of uterine activity are amenable to treatment. Past or current history of infection, presence of membrane rupture and stage of cervical dilatation must be considered.
- The most experienced obstetrician on duty should assess all suspected preterm labours. Accurate diagnosis and proper assessment is essential for correct management. Fetal age, numbers, weight and presentation are significant factors governing outcome. If in-house expertise or facilities are not available, consider transfer to a tertiary hospital.
- Obtain detailed obstetric and medical history from the mother. Identify conditions which contraindicate drug therapy or attempts to stop preterm labour or delivery.
- Management of preterm labour, particularly at the extremely preterm periods of gestation, can leave significant psychosocial consequences

for the parents. There is also clinical risk of mortality and morbidity for the mother from prolonged tocolysis, haemorrhage (more than 1000 ml), thrombosis and sepsis if surgery is performed. Some 6% of uterine scars dehisce in future pregnancies after a classical caesarean section.

- Senior neonatologists and obstetricians must counsel parents fully (preferably at a joint meeting) about complications, likelihood of neonatal survival and eventual outcome. Parents must be made aware that expected outcome can change after delivery depending on the baby's condition at birth, presence of infection, sex of the baby and results of neonatal care such as residue lung disease or intracranial lesions. Respect the parents' informed choice. They have to live with the consequences.

Preterm labour at 23–26 completed weeks

Preterm labour and delivery at these extremely early gestations present both ethical and clinical challenges. The following current evidence will help counselling:

- Between 23 and 24 weeks every extra day increases survival by 3%. From 24–26 weeks there is a 2% increase.
- Increase in birthweight especially between 600 g and 800 g enhances survival.
- Females and Afro-Caribbean compared to Caucasian babies have survival advantages.
- Pregnancy complications leading to delivery at these extremely early gestations do not influence survival before discharge from hospital.
- Singleton babies are more likely to survive compared to twins, especially between 700 and 999 g.
- Overall prevalence of moderate or severe cerebral palsy is 1.5–2.5 per 1000 live births. Below 1500 g at birth the incidence is 50 per 1000. Table 13.2 lists survival rates and incidence of major handicaps such as neuro-developmental deficits with spastic diplegia, hemiplegia, quadriplegia or sensory and intellectual impairment after delivery at extremely early gestations.

Table 13.2 Percentage survival and survival with handicap between gestations 23 weeks and 26 weeks and 6 days

Gestation in weeks	23	24	25	26+6 days
Survival (%)	15	40	50	60
Survivors with handicap (%)	65	35	30	25

- A poorly formed lower uterine segment necessitates use of classical caesarean section for delivery.
- Before 26 completed weeks of gestation there is no evidence to suggest benefit or danger for corticosteroid administration. A full course of corticosteroids (two doses of 12 mg dexamethasone 12 hours apart) for fetuses between 28 and 34 weeks gestation reduces mortality, incidence of respiratory distress and intraventricular haemorrhage. Use of thyrotrophin-releasing hormone is not recommended.
- Beta-adrenergic agonists (e.g. ritodrine) are currently not indicated before 23 weeks gestation. There is more risk than benefit for ritodrine use in twin or high multiple pregnancies between 23 weeks and 26 weeks and 6 days.
- Neonatal outcome is not improved by prophylactic antibiotic therapy at this early gestation.
- Before 23 weeks in utero transfer is seldom indicated. Perform caesarean section when there is maternal indication. Compassionate care only for the baby is acceptable.
- Between 23 weeks and 26 weeks and 6 days transfer if clinically appropriate for delivery at a tertiary hospital. Perform caesarean section only after full discussion with the parents.
- Delayed cord clamping brings likely benefit by reduced need for transfusion.
- An experienced neonatologist must attend delivery. The parents' wishes must be considered in neonatal care immediately after delivery. The condition at delivery significantly affects outcome.

Cervical cerclage

Emergency cerclage has been performed for gestations as late as 26 completed weeks with intact membranes and cervical dilatation between 3 and 10 cm with reported perinatal survival of 45–63%. When compared with conservative management with bed rest, the incidence of infection, need for caesarean section and perinatal mortality appeared similar. A successful outcome is more likely before 20 weeks gestation, and for cervical dilatations of less than 4 cm, when the C reactive protein is less than 4 mg/dl and the white cell count is below 14 000. Cervical cerclage requires:

- Intact membranes and no uterine contractions.
- Counsel mother about risks, for example infection; possible outcome of procedure, for example fetal membrane rupture; and potential for success.
- Commence tocolytics 2 hours before surgery. Tocolytics should be continued for 24 hours after surgery. Whether amnioreduction before cerclage improves success rates remains controversial.
- Place mother in a slightly head down position for surgery. General anaesthesia with halothane or tocolytics and spinal anaesthesia help relax the uterus.
- Place sponge forceps at positions 3, 6, 9 and 12 of the cervix to provide counter traction. Bulging membranes are reduced by gentle traction on all four sponge forceps followed by gentle insertion of a lubricated gauze roll through the cervix. Alternatively, insert a Foley's catheter and inflate the balloon (Fig. 13.1).
- Once the membranes are reduced insert cervical sutures (usually in form of a tape) as high as is feasible. Note position of bladder and ureters. Take interrupted bites above placement of the sponge forceps and tie the knot at 3 or 9 o'clock for easy access. Do not tie beneath bladder as the knot will cause irritation.

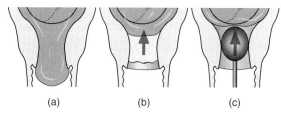

(a)   (b)   (c)

Figure 13.1 Reduction of bulging membranes (a), by gauze roll (b), or by inflated balloon (c).

- Following surgery prescribe bed rest for 24–48 hours. Ambulate when there is no uterine irritability.
- There is a place for an abdominal approach for cervical cerclage.
- Before leaving hospital advise to watch for discharge, vaginal infection and onset of labour.

Preterm labour – antibiotics and infection

Vaginal microorganisms such as *group B streptococci, Listeria monocytogenes* and *Gardnerella vaginalis* are associated with preterm labour and preterm premature membrane rupture (PPROM). Current understanding is:

- Use of antibiotics showed significant advantage after PPROM in maternal (e.g. chorioamnionitis or endometritis) and neonatal outcome (respiratory distress syndrome, intraventricular haemorrhage, sepsis and cerebral palsy).
- Whether antibiotic treatment of vaginal microorganisms prevents preterm labour or PPROM remains controversial. There are, however, reports of infection as a cause in 40% of spontaneous preterm labour and administration of intravenous antibiotics have delayed delivery. The ORACLE II randomized trial (Kenyon et al 2001) advised against routine prescription of antibiotics without clinical evidence of infection.
- For preterm premature rupture of membranes antibiotic therapy can delay delivery for 1 week and reduce maternal and neonatal infection, hence it should be used especially between 23 and 26 completed weeks (see below).
- Around 10–15% of mothers carry *group B haemolytic streptococci*. A history of fever and 'flu-like' illness may indicate *Listeria monocytogenes* infection. If infection is suspected prescribe ampicillin (2 g statum and 1 g 6-hourly intravenously for 10 days or until delivery). Add metronidazole (1 g per rectum 3 times a day) if chorioamnionitis is likely. If penicillin is contraindicated substitute ampicillin with a cephalosporin, for example cefotaxime (1 g intravenously 8-hourly). Note there is 5–10% cross sensitivity with cephalosporins. Alternatively erythromycin 250 mg (drug of choice, see below) in divided doses can be used. Notify the neonatologist.

PRETERM PREMATURE MEMBRANE RUPTURE (PPROM)

The incidence of spontaneous rupture of fetal membranes before 37 weeks gestation is around 3–6%. Contributory factors include infection (e.g. *group B haemolytic streptococcus*), polyhydramnios or collagen defect. Some 30–40% of preterm labour is preceded by membrane rupture. This complication is the most significant factor for likelihood of preterm labour and delivery (Table 13.3). Once membranes rupture, 50% of mothers will labour spontaneously in 24 hours and 80% will commence labour in 48 hours. When suspected PPROM presents:

- Perform speculum examination with strict aseptic technique. A pool of liquor in the posterior fornix is a classic sign. Fetal fibronectin testing is expensive. A negative test suggests labour is unlikely but even if the test is positive some 80% need not deliver in the near future. If membranes are ruptured exclude cord prolapse.
- Take swabs for bacterial culture. Chorioamnionitis is often present, threatening wound infection and neonatal sepsis.
- Look out for signs of herpetic infection.
- Chorioamnionitis is associated with maternal tachycardia with or without fever (pyrexia may be absent in gram negative septicaemia). There is uterine tenderness when palpated

Table 13.3 Effect of listed conditions on likelihood of preterm delivery following preterm labour

Factor	Calculated weight	Weighting given in preterm labour score
Membranes	1.45	1.5
'Show'	1.17	1
Dilatation	1.38	1.5
Contributory factors	1.05	1
Contradictions	0.71	–

and evidence of fetal tachycardia or ominous fetal heart rate changes. An offensive vaginal discharge may be evident. When infection is established consider delivery whatever the gestation. Some 10% of fetuses will be infected.

- For gestations of 32 or more weeks with confirmed membrane rupture, risk of cord prolapse and infection outweigh preterm delivery. Allow preterm labour to continue if there are no contraindications (e.g. footling breech which necessitates caesarean section). In the absence of uterine contractions and when cervical conditions are not favourable for induction of labour, adopt conservative management (hospitalization, bed rest and antibiotics).
- Uterine infection, if not present, will occur after 4 hours of membrane rupture. Deliver by caesarean section if active herpetic lesions are evident and membrane rupture is less than 4 hours.
- Between gestations of 27 and 32 weeks, adopt conservative management if there is no uterine activity. Prescribe corticosteroids. With preterm labour and no contraindications, tocolytics and antibiotics can gain an extra week and reduce maternal and fetal morbidity.
- Erythromycin 250 mg 4 times daily for 10 days can prolong pregnancies and benefit neonatal outcome. Coamoxiclav is not recommended because of its association with increase in occurrence of neonatal necrotizing enterocolitis.

PRETERM LABOUR AND TOCOLYTICS

- Beta-adrenergic agonists such as salbutamol, terbutaline and especially ritodrine are the most commonly used tocolytics. Magnesium sulphate and prostaglandin synthase antagonist are not licensed for use. Prostaglandin synthase antagonists cross the placenta and exert serious fetal vascular side effects such as closure of the ductus arteriosus.
- Exclude contraindications for stopping preterm labour and use of drugs (e.g. maternal heart disease).
- Before 26 weeks and 6 days use of beta agonists may confer more harm than benefit.

> **Box 13.1**   Use of beta-sympathomimetics
>
> - Can delay delivery for 48 hours.
> - No effect on perinatal mortality or morbidity.
> - Mother's heart rate must not exceed 130–140 BPM.
> - Mother must be closely monitored. Hypotension can result.
> - Monitor fluid balance. If pulmonary oedema is diagnosed stop treatment and prescribe diuretics.
> - Do not prescribe beta-sympathomimetics to mothers with cardiac disease. The increased cardiac output can cause myocardial ischaemia.
> - Diabetes will need adjustment of blood sugar levels since carbohydrate metabolism is affected.
> - Beta-sympathomimetics can cross the placenta to produce similar effects in the fetus (e.g. fetal tachycardia) as in the mother.
> - Some 14% of mothers stop treatment because of side effects such as tachycardia, dyspnoea, palpitation or chest pain.
> - Oxytocin antagonist is a possible safer alternative.

- Strict surveillance for beta agonist usage is essential. Careful fluid balance, avoidance of intravenous saline, monitoring with electrocardiography and frequent auscultation of lung basis to exclude pulmonary oedema are recommended. Box 13.1 gives guidelines on the use of beta-sympathomimetics.
- The aim is to prevent delivery for 24–48 hours to allow corticosteroid therapy to enhance fetal lung maturity. Significant fetal benefit is not demonstrated (perinatal mortality, morbidity and increase in birthweight).
- Tocolytics such as selective Cox II cyclo-oxygenase enzyme inhibitors and pro drug prostaglandin synthase inhibitors with predominantly maternal effect may be potentially useful. The oxytocin antagonist Tractocile (atosiban) is licensed for treatment of preterm labour. This competitive inhibitor of oxytocin is as effective as beta agonist in delaying delivery for 48 hours and possibly safer for the mother, but neonatal outcome is the same.

General guidance for preterm labour and delivery management is presented in Box 13.2.

PRETERM DELIVERY

Preterm labour and delivery remain serious complications with significant sequelae for mothers

---

Box 13.2   Management of preterm labour and delivery

- Clinical assessment by most experienced obstetrician on duty when mother presents with possible preterm labour. Perform sterile speculum examination. Take swabs for microscopy and culture. Define cervical status. Address reasons for admission if diagnosis is not confirmed. Follow plan in Table 13.1.
- Check medical and obstetric history. If delivery is not imminent determine gestational age and clinical status. Perform ultrasound scan. Note contraindications to stop preterm delivery and exclude risk of medical treatment with tocolytics. Consider need for in utero transfer. Tocolysis is not likely to succeed if labour is established and the cervix is ≥5 cm dilated (Table 13.1).
- Between 27 and 34 weeks gestation and with no contraindications to stop labour prescribe tocolytics and corticosteroids. Arrange transfer if indicated and safe. Discuss with parents and neonatologists to obtain an agreed mode for delivery if tocolysis fails.

- For preterm labour between 23 weeks and 26 weeks and 6 days gestation note earlier advice. Respect the parental wishes. An experienced neonatologist must attend delivery to determine if active resuscitation is appropriate. External cardiac massage and adrenaline need not improve survival. Request for neonatologist to attend delivery for babies less than 23 weeks gestation is principally to support the parents.
- Monitor the fetal heart rate continuously by ultrasound throughout labour. Prompt response is required to prevent hypoxic damage of these susceptible fetuses.
- An epidural block provides the best form of analgesia and obviates need for opiates which aggravate neonatal respiratory problems.
- Do not use the Ventouse. An episiotomy can facilitate delivery. Forceps are designed for a term baby. A small Wrigley's forceps may be more appropriate for assisted vaginal delivery.

---

and their newborns. The informed views of the parent, neonatologists and obstetricians must be considered, preferably at a joint meeting, to determine an agreed best plan of management. Established preterm labour seldom responds to tocolytics for any length of time, hence the main focus must be on the most competent site and most suitable mode of delivery for best results. Where necessary, appropriate and safe in utero transfer is preferred. There is a place for compassionate care for the extremely preterm baby, especially if delivered in poor condition.

REFERENCES

Kenyon S L, Taylor D J, Tarnow-Mordi 2001 Broad spectrum antibiotics for spontaneous preterm labour: the ORACLE II randomised trial. Lancet 357: 979–988

FURTHER READING

Anon A 1995 Effect of corticosteroids for fetal maturation on perinatal outcomes. NIH Consensus Development Panel on the effect of corticosteroids for fetal maturation on the perinatal outcomes. Journal of American Medical Association 273: 413–418

Canadian Preterm Labour Investigators' Group 1992 Treatment of pre-term labour with the beta-adrenergic agonist ritodrine. New England Journal of Medicine 327: 308–312

Goodwin T M, Palenzuela G J, Silver H, Creasy G (Datospian Study Group) 1996 Dose ranging study of the oxytocin antagonist atosiban in the treatment of pre-term labour. Obstetrics and Gynecology 88: 331–336

Finnstrom O, Olausson P O, Sedin G et al 1997 The Swedish national prospective study on extremely low birthweight (ELBW) infants. Incidence, mortality, morbidity and survival in relation to level of care. Acta Paediatrica 86: 503–511

Kenyon S L, Taylor D J, Tarnow-Mordi W 2001 Broad spectrum antibiotics for preterm, pre-labour rupture of fetal membranes; the ORACLE I randomised trial. Lancet 357: 979–988

The World Wide Atosiban A versus Beta Agonists Study Group 2001 Effectiveness and safety of the oxytocin antagonist atosiban versus beta adrenergic agonists in the treatment of pre-term labour. British Journal of Obstetrics and Gynaecology 108: 133–142

14

Abnormal labour

D. Liu, M. Whittle

Spontaneous onset of labour followed by efficient uterine activity and delivery after around 8 hours for multiparous and 12–14 hours for primiparous mothers is accepted as normal. Labour complicated by problems of uterine contractility or integrity (powers), adequacy of the pelvis (passage), and fetal complication (passenger) is considered abnormal.

ABNORMAL UTERINE ACTIVITY

False labour (spurious labour)

Braxton Hicks or practice contractions may be exceptionally uncomfortable or of longer duration, thus giving the impression that labour has started. On the other hand repeated episodes of false labour or spurious labour can signify fetal compromise and the need for early delivery to avoid fetal death.

Management

- Assess the mother to establish whether or not she is in labour. Observe contraction strength and frequency; check cervix on admission and review 1–2 hours later. If the cervix is <4 cm and there is no dilatation over the observation period, she is either in the latent phase of labour or not in labour. Assess fetal wellbeing using a 20 minute CTG. If deemed not in active labour and fetus is satisfactory, she may go to the ward to await events. If appropriate some mothers may even go home.
- The presence of risk factors, e.g. abnormalities in the pregnancy or a non-reassuring CTG,

indicate the need for close surveillance with consideration to augment or induce labour.

- Mothers should be fully informed, contribute to plans for their care and be aware of the reasons for the steps taken.

Precipitate labour and delivery

Labour resulting in delivery less than 2 hours after onset of uterine contractions is accepted as rapid or precipitate. Dangers include delivery in an unsuitable or non-sterile environment with risk of fetal and maternal trauma.

Precipitate labour and delivery are likely in the following conditions.

- When there is little resistance to delivery. With an effaced cervix 3 cm or more dilated and the presenting part engaged and well applied, little harm is likely if labour is properly conducted in an appropriate environment. Mothers with a history of precipitate labours should be admitted around 38 weeks for induction of labour to control the situation.
- Rapid labour may follow sensitivity to or excessive use of oxytocics. The fetus is pushed rapidly through the birth canal by strong frequent uterine contractions. Fetal hypoxia and trauma together with soft tissue damage of the birth canal are likely. This should not happen in well conducted labours.

Management

- Anticipate the situation from obstetric history. Mothers for oxytocin stimulation must be carefully selected. This is particularly important in the grand multipara or those mothers with a history of short labours.
- Anticipate the condition if pelvic findings suggest the likelihood of rapid labour.
- The mother's and fetal condition must be closely monitored. A midwife must be in attendance to supervise labour.
- Myometrial sensitivity to syntocinon is enhanced after prostaglandin usage.
- Following delivery, examine the soft tissue of the birth canal for possible damage.

Sudden cessation of labour

When labour stops suddenly suspect uterine rupture. Uterine rupture is usually, but not always, preceded by evidence of fetal distress and continuous lower abdominal pain.

Management

- Confirm the diagnosis.
- Assess maternal condition, treat if shocked.
- The globular outline of the uterus is lost, fetal parts may be readily palpable, the fetal heart sounds may be absent, lie may not be longitudinal.

Box 14.1   Uterine rupture

Classification
Rupture may be incomplete (intact peritoneum) or complete (uterine cavity communicates directly with peritoneum cavity). This complication occurs in between 1 in 140 and 1 in 300 labours with a uterine scar.

Associations
- Previous uterine damage or surgery, e.g. myomectomy which encroached into uterine cavity, hysterotomy and perforations.
- Caesarean sections, particularly classical sections (may rupture before onset of labour). Multiple sections or sections with inadvertent extension or need for an inverted T incision (Ch. 17). History of infection may mean poor healing and a weaker scar.
- Obstructed labour.
- Oxytocic usage. The very unfavourable cervix, previous lower segment caesarean section and oxytocic augmentation in multiparous women require careful assessment and close observation.
- Prostaglandin pessaries should be used with caution when priming a cervix in the presence of a previous caesarean scar.
- Instrumental delivery, e.g. rotation forceps.
- Intrauterine manipulations, e.g. internal podalic version for assisted breech delivery.
    This complication contributes to maternal and high perinatal mortality. Prevention by attention to above is important.

Diagnosis
See Chapter 17.

Subsequent care
- Provide opportunity for counselling to explain reasons for this traumatic incident.
- Elective caesarean section and close antenatal surveillance is mandatory if further pregnancies are allowed when the uterus is salvaged.

- Cross-match blood, summon an experienced anaesthetist and senior obstetrician.
- Perform emergency laparotomy.
- If repair of the uterus is not possible proceed to hysterectomy. There is a place for subtotal hysterectomy in this situation.

Box 14.1 gives further information on uterine rupture.

PROLONGED LABOUR

Labour is prolonged if it lasts more than 24 hours. This concept is dangerous if it suggests the mistaken connotation that labour can continue for 24 hours before delay is diagnosed. Labour should be considered prolonged once it lags behind the normal partogram by 2–3 hours. This definition draws attention earlier to development of abnormality.

Prolonged labour is due to:

- abnormal contractions (powers)
- deficient/delayed cervical dilatation (passage)
- abnormal descent of the presenting part of the fetus (passenger).

Abnormal contractions (powers)

Infrequent weak contractions (hypotonic uterine activity)

Most likely reason is misdiagnosis of labour. It has been said that the overstretched uterus does not labour well but evidence for this is thin.

Management

- Assess the mother's status, support her morale and correct ketoacidosis.
- If there are no contraindications (exclude disproportion and malpresentation), augment labour by amniotomy with or without intravenous oxytocics.
- Maintain close surveillance.

Frequent strong contractions (hypertonic contractions)

These can follow the inappropriate use of oxytocics. Prolonged labour associated with strong contractions is seen principally in multiparous mothers with disproportion. The practised uterus mounts an increased effort to overcome the obstruction. The resultant frequent strong contractions and increased uterine tone distress both the mother and fetus. If allowed to continue tetanic uterine activity can occur. A retraction ring denoting the junction between the strong contracting upper uterine segment and the overstretched lower segment is observed as a late sign of imminent uterine rupture.

Management

- An abnormal fetal heart rate is often an early sign and should alert the attendant to the problem.
- Exclude overstimulation by oxytocics.
- Caesarean section is indicated for tetanic contractions and an overstretched lower segment. This should be considered even if the fetus is dead. Destructive operations for a dead fetus increase the risk of uterine rupture.
- If the situation is less acute, reassess presentation and position of the presenting part of the fetus. The mode of delivery will depend on the findings and include trial of forceps, rotation forceps or more usually caesarean section.
- Excessive uterine activity can sometimes be reduced using salbutamol by inhalation for immediate effect.

Incoordinate uterine activity

The pacemaker for myometrial activity is normally situated at the cornu of the uterus. When pacemaker activity develops at alternative sites and interrupts fundal dominance, irregular uterine contractions are produced and incoordinate uterine activity results. Incoordinate uterine activity produces poor uterine propulsive effort, increased uterine tone and intermittent painful strong uterine contractions (Fig. 14.1). This is usually, but not exclusively, a condition of primiparous mothers where an element of disproportion is present. This condition is more likely if the mother is frightened, distressed or anxious as in a first labour, particularly if she is over the age of 35 years.

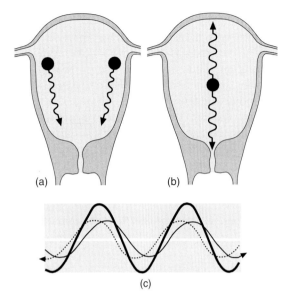

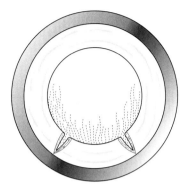

Figure 14.2 Cervical incisions.

Figure 14.1 Fundal dominance with (a) normal pacemaker activity, (b) ectopic pacemaker and incoordinated uterine activity, (c) schematic illustration of ectopic pacemaker activity resulting in high amplitude and attenuated contraction waves of incoordinated activity.

Management

- Reassure the mother, sedate if appropriate and prescribe analgesia. Epidural anaesthesia is particularly effective.
- More than 50% of these mothers may require assisted delivery. Group and save blood.
- Re-examine the mother to exclude absolute disproportion.
- If appropriate, rupture the membranes and apply direct fetal heart rate monitoring.
- Prescribe intravenous oxytocics if there is no contraindication to further labour. The use of oxytocics overrides pacemaker influence.
- Deliver by caesarean section if there is no progress after 2–4 hours of oxytocic therapy or if fetal distress develops.

Deficient/delayed cervical dilatation (passage)

Poor cervical dilatation reflects or contributes to the slow progress of labour. The following points should be noted:

- The cervix dilates less well if the presenting part of the fetus is poorly applied.
- Occurs in 5% of primigravida. This can be associated with poor cervical response to pregnancy changes. Assisted delivery or caesarean section is likely.
- Strong labour with poor descent can produce an oedematous cervix and gives the impression that dilatation is regressing.
- Poor dilatation can reflect weak or incoordinated uterine activity.
- Poor dilatation can be associated with disproportion.
- A scarred or fibrotic cervix (following cerclage or cone biopsy) may not dilate despite the descent of the presenting part to the introitus. If there is failure to dilate beyond 5 cm or more, incise the cervix 2 cm at the 5 and 7 o'clock regions and deliver by forceps (Fig. 14.2). Cervical incisions are seldom performed because further extension during delivery with resultant haemorrhage and damage to the lower uterine segment can occur. Do not incise if the cervix is not thinned out; deliver by caesarean section.

Abnormal descent

Any condition that hinders descent will prolong labour. Obstruction to descent is due to the following:

- Obstruction by a mass or tumour outside the uterus, for example an ovarian cyst. Malpresentation and malposition are usual. Obstruction can be at any level, such as the pelvic brim or upper half of the pelvis. This complication should be identified before the onset of labour. Delivery is by caesarean section. An experienced obstetrician is required to conduct or supervise any additional surgery.
- Masses such as fibroids arising from the uterus or cervix can interfere with descent of the fetus. Occasionally, after a lengthy labour when little residual liquor is present, the uterus may be wrapped tightly around the fetus, preventing descent. Caesarean section is required. A possible exception is where forceps delivery is prevented by tonic uterine contraction. When this occurs the uterus can be relaxed by amyl nitrate, salbutamol inhalation or halothane administration to allow vaginal delivery.
- The presence of an unsuspected degree of placenta praevia.
- Disproportion. This term describes the situation where the proportions or diameters of the pelvis are inadequate for the passage of the fetus. This terminology describes inadequacy of the pelvis to accommodate the fetal head, which has the largest diameter and is least compressible. Cephalopelvic disproportion is a relative concept. A larger than normal baby can produce disproportion in a pelvis which is of normal size. This concept is particularly relevant in multiparous labours. The fetus may be greater in size in subsequent pregnancies so previous spontaneous delivery should not encourage complacency. Alternatively, a small or preterm baby may deliver with ease through a small or contracted pelvis. Disproportion may arise at any stage of labour or at any site along the pelvic canal. It is, however, usual to notice disproportion at the pelvic brim (inlet disproportion), at the level of the ischial spine (mid pelvic disproportion at the plane of least diameter) and at the pelvic outlet (outlet disproportion). Labour is prolonged whenever disproportion is present.

Management

- Perform vaginal examination to assess cervical status, station of the presenting part of the fetus, presence of caput and adequacy of the pelvis.
- Request erect lateral pelvimetry. Additional information concerning the shape of the sacrum and possible reasons for inlet disproportion may be obtained.
- Perform a caesarean section if absolute disproportion is diagnosed at the inlet, mid pelvis or outlet. Absolute disproportion is present whenever any pelvic diameter is smaller than the biparietal diameter. For the average fetus a diameter of 9.5 cm is not adequate.
- Inlet disproportion is associated with a flat pelvis, spondylolisthesis, sacralization of the fifth lumbar vertebra, pelvic deformity (rickets, osteomalacia), pelvic fracture or congenital defects (Naegele's or Robert's pelvis). If absolute disproportion is not evident (fetal head overlaps symphysis when an attempt is made to direct the head into the pelvis) and there is no contraindication to further labour, observe closely and review after 2 hours. Cord prolapse is a threat when the presenting part of the fetus is poorly applied. Delivery by caesarean section is usual.
- Mid pelvic disproportion. Both the short, stocky, obese, hirsute mother and the tall athletic mother with boyish hips are susceptible. Malposition is common. If conditions are suitable for further labour, review after an interval of 2 hours. Deliver by caesarean section if there is no progress. If the cervix is fully dilated and there is no absolute disproportion, Ventouse or forceps delivery by an experienced obstetrician may be attempted after correction of malposition.
- Outlet disproportion. This presents classically as delay in the second stage. The cervix is fully dilated with the presenting part below the midplane. A trial of forceps is acceptable if absolute disproportion is excluded. Outlet disproportion must be excluded in a breech delivery.

Problems with the passenger

The third group of causes for failure to progress is due to problems with the passenger (fetus/fetuses). There are four main factors:

1. fetus too big
2. malposition
3. malpresentation
4. fetal abnormality.

It is essential, when faced with poor progress, that these factors are excluded. Malposition can sometimes be corrected by the use of oxytocin but its injudicious use in the other situations may result in uterine rupture.

Fetal abnormality includes conjoined twins or tumours, for example cystic hygromas. In contemporary practice most of these are identified antenatally by ultrasound scanning. In twin labour, consider 'locking' when there is failure of descent despite ideal conditions. Caesarean section is usually required. The risk is highest when the first twin is breech.

Fetal abnormality also includes growth retardation. See Box 14.2 for procedure in cases of intrauterine growth restriction.

CONSEQUENCES OF PROLONGED LABOUR

Fetus

The consequences for the fetus include trauma, acidosis, hypoxic damage, infection and increased perinatal mortality and morbidity.

Mother

The consequences for the mother are reduced morale, exhaustion, dehydration, acidosis, infection and risk of uterine rupture. The need for surgical intervention increases mortality and morbidity. Ketoacidosis by itself can result in poor uterine activity and prolonged labour.

General management

- Anticipate likelihood of this complication before the onset of labour or at the initial assessment in the labour suite.

Box 14.2 Intrauterine growth restriction

- Confirm diagnosis from obstetric history and ultrasound measurements. Umbilical artery Doppler waveform and cardiotocograph trace can indicate impaired fetal–placental perfusion. Late onset growth restriction may be associated with normal umbilical artery Doppler findings despite fetal compromise because of compensatory mechanisms.
- Determine if the fetus is anatomical and chromosomally normal. Fetal weight less than 500 g after 26 weeks, presence of reverse end diastolic flow velocity in umbilical arteries, umbilical vein pulsations and cardiotocographic fetal heart rate decelerations forewarn of poor prognosis.
- Review situation with parents and neonatologist. Offer counselling where appropriate.
- Determine mode of delivery. Consider past obstetric history, past labour patterns and presenting cervical conditions. Before 34 weeks of pregnancy presence of severe fetal compromise and anticipated viability justifies elective caesarean section. Use intravenous oxytocin to induce labour (starting at 2–4 mu/min). This is similar to performing a contraction stress test. Appearance of decelerations necessitates delivery by caesarean section.
- Prostaglandin is not contraindicated when there is no Doppler or fetal heart rate signs of compromise.
- Perform caesarean section if induction of labour is not successful.
- Fetal heart rate monitoring and close surveillance is mandatory during labour if growth restriction is suspected.
- Use the lower midline vertical uterine incision for delivery for fetuses less than 750 g if lower uterine segment is poorly formed. Monitor fetal heart rate till just before skin incision.
- Consider general anaesthesia which is associated with less fetal acidaemia.
- In preterm growth restricted fetuses presence of pregnancy hypertension confers advantage with reduced perinatal mortality. Perinatal mortality rises significantly after 40 weeks of pregnancy.
- A neonatologist must attend delivery as these babies have impaired metabolic adaptation such as poor response to hypoglycaemic stress, increased risk of necrotizing enterocolitis, and respiratory distress syndrome.

- Determine the cause of prolonged labour. Treat correctable causes.
- Determine if there is justification for further continuation of labour. Fetal or maternal compromise precludes further labour.
- Continuing labour must be closely monitored. Support mother's morale and include her and her partner in discussion of the likely outcome.

- Anticipate the possibility of a caesarean section (required for 80% of mothers not responding to oxytocics).

TRIAL OF LABOUR

All labour can be considered a trial. The term trial of labour is reserved for situations where possible complications of labour are anticipated. The trial assesses the adequacy of the pelvis and the ability of the fetus or mother to withstand labour.

Contraindications

- Absolute disproportion.
- Malpresentations such as face and brow.
- Breech presentation. The trunk is the smaller or more compressible part of the fetus. The dangerous situation where the body is delivered with entrapment of the larger fetal head can occur.
- Fetal compromise.
- Maternal complications such as severe pre-eclampsia or severe cardiac disease.
- A uterus already weakened, for example by previous surgery or caesarean section.

Requirements

- Contraindications must be excluded.
- Presence of regular effective uterine contractions. The cautious augmentation of uterine activity by intravenous oxytocics may be required. The trial examines the outcome of contractions. It is not a trial to determine if contractions can be generated or maintained. If possible await spontaneous onset of labour.
- Rupture membranes once the fetal head engages and apply direct fetal heart rate monitoring.
- Close fetal and maternal surveillance is necessary.
- Assessment at 2–4 hour intervals should be made, preferably by the same person.
- There should be adequate analgesia.

- General anaesthesia and surgery may be required. Adjust oral intake and cross-match blood.
- Supportive nursing and full discussion of the situation with the mother must be maintained.

Failed trial of labour

The trial must be abandoned when:

- fetal distress develops
- maternal distress or complications arise
- there is no progress after 2–4 hours despite adequate uterine contractions.

If the anticipated problem is limited to the pelvic outlet and instrumental delivery is considered, the term trial of forceps or Ventouse is used. Delivery is by caesarean section if the trial of labour or trial of instrumental delivery fails. Caesarean section is required for subsequent pregnancies if the fetal size is the same or larger.

TRIAL OF SCAR OR VAGINAL DELIVERY

This term is used when vaginal delivery is considered after a previous lower segment caesarean section or, on occasion, a hysterotomy where the midline incision is sited in the lower half of the uterus.

Contraindications

- Previous classical caesarean section.
- History of uterine damage or plastic reconstruction.
- Suspicion of disproportion.
- History of complications (e.g. infection) which might have affected healing after previous caesarean section or uterine surgery.
- Uterine tenderness when the uterine scar is palpated.

Requirements

Many obstetricians are loath to allow vaginal delivery after any caesarean section. Caesarean section is not without risk and when conditions are satisfactory vaginal delivery can be safer and provide the mother with an experience of normal childbirth. In less than ideal conditions attempts at vaginal delivery can result in uterine rupture. It is, therefore, important that:

- an experienced obstetrician assesses and decides on the mode of delivery;
- the pelvic diameters must be ideal;
- labour is conducted in a properly equipped environment;
- close surveillance of both fetal and maternal conditions is maintained;
- all attending staff are aware of the risks and signs of uterine rupture;

- any expression of increased or continuous pain must be investigated, particularly when epidural analgesia is used. Scar tenderness necessitates suspension of the trial. Deliver by caesarean section;
- a short second stage is imposed. Avoid excessive pushing by performing an episiotomy and the early use of instrumental delivery;
- an experienced obstetrician must supervise or conduct delivery.

The uterine scar may be weakened after each vaginal delivery. Repeated vaginal delivery after previous caesarean section must be conducted with extreme caution.

FURTHER READING

Adamson S L 1999 Arterial pressure, vascular input impedance, and resistance as determinants of pulsatile blood flow in the umbilical artery. European Journal of Obstetrics, Gynecology and Reproductive Biology 84: 119–125

Alfirevic Z, Neilson J P 1995 Doppler ultrasonography in high risk pregnancies: systematic review with meta-analysis. American Journal of Obstetrics and Gynecology 172: 1379–1387

Caldeyro-Barcia R, Alvarez H, Poserro J J 1955 Normal and abnormal uterine contractions in labour. Triangle 2: 41

CESDI, 5th Annual Report 1998 Maternal and Child Health Consortium, London

Chang T C, Robson F C, Spencer J A, Gallivan S 1994 Prediction of perinatal morbidity at term in small fetuses: comparison of fetal growth and Doppler ultrasound. British Journal of Obstetrics and Gynaecology 101: 422–427

Divon M Y, Ajglund B, Niselo H et al 1998 Fetal and neonatal mortality in the post term pregnancy: the impact of gestational age and fetal growth restriction. American Journal of Obstetrics and Gynecology 178: 726–731

Fairweather D V I, Stewart A L 1983 How to deliver the under-1500 gram infant. Reid's controversy in obstetrics and gynaecology, 3rd edn. Saunders, Philadelphia, London, p 154

Friedman E A 1954 The graphic analysis of labour. American Journal of Obstetrics and Gynecology 68: 1569

Kiserud T, Eik-Nes S H, Vlaas H G et al 1994 Ductus venous blood flow velocity and the umbilical circulation in the seriously growth retarded fetus. Ultrasound Obstetrics and Gynaecology 4: 109–114

Phelan J P, Clarke S L, Daiz M A, Paul R H 1987 Vaginal birth after Caesarean. American Journal of Obstetrics and Gynecology 157: 1510–1515

Piper J M, Xenakis E M, McFarland M et al 1996 Do growth retarded premature infants have different rates of perinatal morbidity and mortality than appropriately grown premature infants? Obstetrics and Gynecology 87: 169–174

Steward K S, Philpott R H 1980 Fetal response to cephalopelvic disproportion. British Journal of Obstetrics and Gynaecology 87: 641

Studd J 1975 The partographic control of labour. Clinics in Obstetrics and Gynecology 2: 127

Tyson J E, Kennedy K, Broyles S, Rosenfeld C R 1995 The small for gestational age infant: accelerated or delayed pulmonary maturation? Increased or decreased survival? Paediatrics 95: 534–538

15

Induction and augmentation of labour

D. Liu, S. Mukhopadhyay,
S. Arulkumaran

Induction of labour is a process for initiation of uterine activity to achieve vaginal delivery. Induction rates between 10% and 25% reflect current policies, referral patterns and sometimes mothers' choices. Labour is initiated to benefit principally the mother, the fetus or both and as an elective prophylactic procedure.

INDUCTION OF LABOUR AS THERAPY

This is considered for the following reason:

- when it is safer for the mother not to continue pregnancy
- when the fetus is less at risk if delivered or when both mother and fetus benefit by delivery.

Close surveillance in labour is mandatory when induction is carried out to address fetal or maternal compromise. If fetal CTG abnormalities develop or labour is not progressing well, early resort to caesarean section is advised. At full cervical dilatation elective or early use of assisted vaginal delivery can be appropriate.

INDICATIONS FOR INDUCTION
Maternal

Medical or obstetric conditions not responding to treatment and which threaten the mother's health, such as heart failure, severe preeclampsia and deteriorating renal function or central nervous system disorders, indicate induction.

Fetal

In the fetus presence of progressive growth retardation, abnormality not compatible with life, or fetal death, are all indications for induction.

Fetus and mother

Induction of labour is also indicated when it would benefit both the mother and fetus, such as in poorly controlled diabetes, following rupture of fetal membranes or when chorioamnionitis is evident. This indication is particularly pertinent in contemporary obstetric practice where women with medical conditions previously not considered suitable for pregnancy are now prepared to accept inherent risks to become mothers.

INDUCTION OF LABOUR AS PROPHYLAXIS

Induction of labour is also considered to anticipate potential complications. Examples are:

- Evidence suggests the fetus is best delivered before 10 days post term (40 complete weeks of pregnancy). Prophylactic induction reduces the incidence of caesarean section, instrumental delivery, fetal compromise during labour and perinatal mortality.
- To achieve better control after previous precipitated labour (labour less than 2 hours).
- To avoid fetal demise in prior unexplained sudden death after fetal maturity.
- To avoid macrosomia and complications of shoulder dystocia especially in a diabetic mother.
- Occasionally induction is considered for logistic or psychosocial reasons such as difficult access to hospital due to distance.

INDUCTION: GENERAL CONSIDERATIONS

- Labour can subject both mother and fetus to stress. If there is significant compromise consider caesarean section as the preferred mode of delivery.

- When advice for induction of labour is declined, close fetal and/or maternal surveillance is essential, e.g. scan for liquor level; twice weekly CTG.
- When induction for fetal or maternal compromise fails, deliver by caesarean section. When failure follows prophylactic indications there is the option to reassess and repeat the process.

CONTRAINDICATIONS TO INDUCTION

Induction of labour should not be considered in the following situations:

- When vaginal delivery is not advised or possible, for example pelvic disproportion, placenta praevia, cord presentation and in the presence of active infection such as genital herpes.
- Uterine contractions can cause uterine rupture after previous classical or inverted T uterine incision, after myomectomy or surgery which extends into the uterine cavity and where lower segment caesarean section is complicated by extension or infection. Review operation notes from previous caesarean sections. Palpate to exclude tenderness over previous lower segment caesarean section scar.
- Induction is contraindicated if labour threatens further compromise for mother and/or fetus.

REQUIREMENTS BEFORE INDUCTION OF LABOUR

- Review medical and obstetric history. Perform clinical examination to exclude contraindications for induction of labour. Ensure mother and partner are fully informed of risk and benefits and consent to the intended programme. Provide written information.
- Perform vaginal examination to assess adequacy of pelvis and determine cervical status. Cervical dilatation, cervical length, consistency, position and station of presenting part are combined into a score, the Bishop's score, often modified to describe cervical status (Fig. 15.1). A low

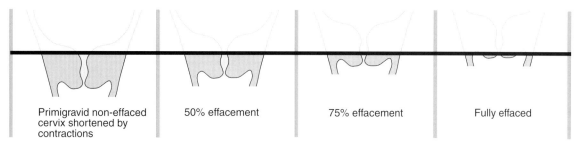

| Primigravid non-effaced cervix shortened by contractions | 50% effacement | 75% effacement | Fully effaced |

Figure 15.1 Cross-section of cervix to illustrate the degree of effacement.

score forewarns of increased likelihood of induction failure and need for cervical preparation or ripening.

- Cervical dilatation exerts twice the influence on successful induction compared with cervical consistency.

PROCESS OF INDUCTION OF LABOUR

Cervical status governs choice for methods to induce labour. A low or unfavourable cervical score necessitates a ripening process for effacement and/or softening of the cervix to facilitate cervical dilatation. This is achieved by drugs, for example prostaglandins, which soften the cervix and produce uterine activity to draw up or create cervical effacement.

Cervical ripening

Pharmacological substances such as prostaglandins are prescribed to prepare or ripen the cervix. The current most clinically acceptable and effective (by 5–10 times) is the prostaglandin E_2 (PGE_2). PGE_2 given intravaginally as a pessary, as water soluble gel or more recently in the form of a slow released hydrogel is also associated with fewer systemic side effects. However, vaginal pH, moisture, temperature and infection can all affect efficacy of the preparation. Do not use obstetric cream for vaginal examination if prostaglandins may be given. Where appropriate membrane sweep is returning as an acceptable procedure for uncomplicated pregnancies over 40 weeks.

Induction of labour

Auscultate fetal heart and perform cardiotocographic trace for 30 minutes. Omit if induction is for fetal demise. If the trace is non-reassuring discuss delivering by caesarean section. There is still a place for admission CTG.

Bishop's score of 4 or less

Administer 2 mg prostaglandin gel into posterior fornix. Repeat with 1 mg in 6 hours if needed. Review by experienced obstetrician 6 hours after second dose. Uterine activity usually starts 1 hour after administration of prostaglandin gel. Pharmacological effect lasts up to 4 hours. Continuous cardiotocographic monitoring is essential. When there is no urgency let mother rest overnight and recommence the programme in the morning. A maximum total dose of 4 mg for primigravidae and 3 mg for multigravidae of PGE_2 is used. Oral or vaginal prostaglandin tablets are alternatives (3 mg PGE_2 6-hourly vaginally and repeat once in 6 hours); with ruptured membranes consider oral prostaglandin or intravenous oxytocin.

Bishop's score between 4 and 7 (favourable cervix)

In primigravidae start with 1 mg prostaglandin gel. Repeat after 6 hours if indicated. Again if labour is not established review by experienced obstetrician 6 hours after second dose. A maximum of 4 mg PGE_2 is advised.

In multigravidae start with 1 mg prostaglandin gel and repeat in 6 hours if required. Review

6 hours after last dose if labour is not established. A maximum of 3 mg is advised.

Uterine hypertonus or hyperstimulation may occur. Close fetal surveillance is essential. Monitor fetal heart rate for at least 60 minutes after inserting prostaglandins. Watch out for signs of uterine rupture when there is a lower segment caesarean section scar. If labour is not established by evening, return mother to ward if appropriate and repeat programme in the morning. If labour ensues recommence fetal heart rate monitoring. Repeat tracing when mother is on the ward. If artificial rupture of membranes (ARM) is not possible after course of prostaglandins review situation with senior obstetrician.

Artificial rupture of fetal membranes (ARM)

With a Bishop's score of 8 or more the cervix is often sufficiently dilated to allow access to the fetal membranes. Options are:

- membrane sweep
- artificial rupture of fetal membranes or amniotomy
- rupture fetal membranes and start syntocinon.

Surgical induction of labour can be achieved by passage of an instrument through the cervical os to artificially rupture the fetal membrane. Drainage of amniotic fluid reduces the size of the uterine cavity and promotes more effective contractions by improving the myometrial length–tension ratio. Prostaglandins are also released from the decidua. Onset of labour usually follows amniotomy in 6–12 hours. This interval before onset of labour is shortened by simultaneous use of intravenous infusion of an oxytocic such as syntocinon.

Technique for low ARM (forewater rupture)

- Make sure mother and her partner give consent (verbal or written) and understand the reasons and steps for the procedure.
- Place mother in a suitable position or in the lithotomy position. Use sterile drapes and an aseptic technique.

- The fetal membranes in front of the presenting part can be ruptured by forceps such as Kocher's forceps or various designs of amniohooks (Fig. 15.2).
- If placenta praevia has not been excluded by ultrasound examination, perform a scan in the labour ward or a formal examination under anaesthesia to palpate the vaginal fornices carefully. Suspect placenta praevia if a thick spongy sensation is felt between the fornices and presenting part of the fetus (Fig. 15.3).
- Insert a finger through the cervical os. Palpate the membranes through the internal os for a distance of 2 cm to exclude pulsating vessels associated with vasa praevia or cord presentation.
- When amniotomy is not contraindicated insert a second finger (index and middle fingers are used). Guide the forceps between the fingers to the membranes (Fig. 15.4). The membranes are picked up by the forceps and ruptured by wiping the index finger over the tip of the forceps. This technique allows good control of the amount of tear and the rate of escape of amniotic fluid. Record quantity and colour of liquor (blood stained, meconium or clear).
- Alternatively introduce an amniohook through the cervix. This is guided to a safe area of the

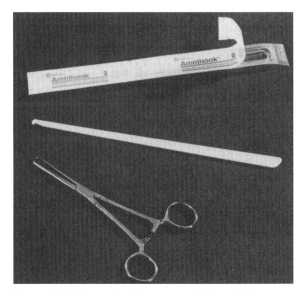

Figure 15.2 Examples of instruments for low ARM.

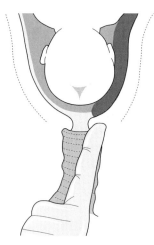

Figure 15.3   Palpation of vaginal fornice to exclude placenta praevia.

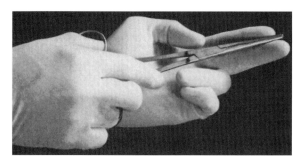

Figure 15.4   Technique for low ARM with Kocher's forceps.

presenting part of the fetus (e.g. away from the fetal face). Approximate amniohook to the membrane by the index finger. The hook is withdrawn to tear the membranes. An advantage of this option is the need for less cervical dilatation but the size of the tear is less predictable.

Infusion of syntocinon

Points to note with syntocinon (synthetic oxytocin) usage are:

- Myometrial sensitivity to oxytocin increases throughout pregnancy and maximum sensitivity is achieved by 34–36 weeks.
- Oxytocin increases both frequency and amplitude of contractions. Use minimal dose which produces adequate uterine contractions. Maximum recommended dose is 20 milliunits per minute.
- Prior treatment with prostaglandins potentiates action of oxytocin. Do not use oxytocin before 6 hours after last dose of PGE_2.
- Oxytocin at 30 international units in 500 ml of normal saline will give 1 milliunit per minute if run at 1 ml per hour.
- Intravenous oxytocin can be titrated to give better control of uterine contractions. Commence infusion using regulated drip set to deliver 2 milliunits per minute and escalate dose at 2.0 milliunits per minute every 30 minutes until contractions lasting 40 seconds recur 4–5 times in every 10 minutes. The dosage schedule is indicated in Box 15.1. Most mothers, however, achieve adequate uterine contractions with 12 milliunits per minute of syntocinon. Once labour is established, maintain the same dose until delivery. Some mothers will continue labour when the dose is reduced to 8 milliunits per minute. Infusion pumps can be used to reduce amount of fluid usage (Fig. 15.5).
- After prolonged use of oxytocin maintain infusion for 1 hour after delivery to minimize rise of atonic postpartum haemorrhage.
- Side effects of syntocinon usage include: uterine hyperstimulation, water retention due to an antidiuretic effect once the dosage exceeds 16 milliunits per minute, and maternal and fetal hyponatraemia. Water toxicity and hyponatraemia can cause maternal headache, nausea, psychosis and convulsions. Fetal adverse effects include lethargy, feeding difficulties, apnoea, cyanotic spells, respiratory distress and convulsions. Neonatal hyperbilirubinaemia is described after oxytocin infusion.

Box 15.1   Concentration of syntocinon

- 2–16 mu/minute is physiological range
- 5–10 mu/minute initiates uterine activity comparable to early labour
- 10–15 mu/minute generates uterine activity similar to late first stage of labour
- 20–25 mu/minute produces activity similar to second stage of labour.

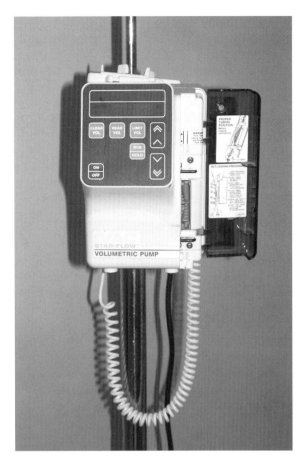

Figure 15.5 Example of infusion pump.

- Start syntocinon once membranes are ruptured, particularly in the primigravida. Close monitoring of mother and fetus is mandatory.
- If ARM is not possible, dispense 1 mg prostaglandin gel if this is appropriate and acceptable to the mother. Monitor fetus as described above.
- Stop oxytocin after 5 hours (5 international units) if labour is not established. Review with senior obstetrician.

RISKS OF INDUCTION

Failed induction

This describes the situation when effective uterine activity is not established or maintained. Failure is less likely for gestations near term or when the Bishop's score is high. When membranes are ruptured there is the risk of infection. Deliver by caesarean section if there is fetal or maternal compromise.

Intrauterine infection

Once membranes rupture intrauterine and fetal infection are more likely. Some mothers, such as those with diabetes, are more susceptible. Following amniotomy only 2.6% of mothers become infected if delivery is achieved within 24 hours compared to 40% when delivery is between 24 and 48 hours. Where possible exclude active vaginal infection such as cervical Herpes and presence of group B streptococcus. Once membranes rupture monitor maternal pulse and fetal heart rate and maternal temperature. Aim to achieve delivery within 24 hours.

Cord prolapse

Incidence of cord prolapse is 0.1–0.5% following membrane rupture. Exclude cord presentation before rupturing membranes. This complication is more likely when the fetal presenting part is not well applied to the cervix or when there is polyhydramnios.

Uterine hyperstimulation

Pharmacological agents used to stimulate uterine activity can lead to excessive amplitude and frequency of contractions. Once the contraction frequency exceeds 5 per 10 minutes uterine activity becomes less efficient. Hyperstimulation follows use of high concentrations of oxytocics or where an individual mother is particularly sensitive to the drug. Hyperstimulation causes fetal hypoxia and threat of uterine rupture, particularly in the grand multipara or in mothers with previous caesarean section scars. Beta-sympathomimetics such as salbutamol by inhalation or other tocolytics such as ritodrine 50–350 (maximum) micrograms per minute or terbutaline, 5–10 micrograms per minute (10 micrograms per minute should seldom be given), can be given intravenously to overcome hyperstimulation.

INDUCTION OF LABOUR – SPECIAL SITUATIONS

Previous caesarean section

- Induction of labour is contraindicated in a uterus with a classical, inverted T or complex extended scar. This statement also applies to situations where the uterine cavity has been entered, such as during myomectomy, when uterine infection has caused poor uterine wound healing and after two previous caesarean sections.
- For high Bishop's scores rupture membranes and titrate uterine activity with intravenous syntocinon.
- For low Bishop's scores administer 1 mg PGE_2 vaginally. The risk of scar dehiscence or rupture varies between 0.7% and 2.2%. Repeat doses of PGE_2 must be balanced against this risk.
- Watch out for signs of scar rupture and fetal distress.

Pre-labour rupture of membranes

Membrane rupture carries risk of cord prolapse and intrauterine infection. Infective morbidity increases after 48 hours. More than 75% of mothers, however, labour spontaneously within 24 hours of membrane rupture.

Take careful history, perform clinical examination to determine presence or absence of uterine activity or uterine tenderness. Confirm the presence of membrane rupture and exclude cord prolapse. Commence cardiotocograph monitoring.

For term fetus (36 completed weeks)

Induce labour immediately if there is threat or evidence of maternal or fetal infection. Deliver by caesarean section if cardiotocograph suggests evidence of fetal compromise.

If there is no risk of complication nor fetal or maternal compromise, discuss options with the mother. Conservative management for 24 hours to await spontaneous onset of labour is acceptable. Induce labour after 24 hours of ruptured membranes.

For 34 weeks of gestation to term

Allow labour to continue. When obstetric risk is present, such as infection or fetal compromise, induce labour or deliver by caesarean section where appropriate.

If conservative management is acceptable take cervical swabs. Transfer to antenatal ward and commence 4-hourly recording of maternal pulse rate and temperature. Check abdomen for tenderness at the same time. Perform twice daily fetal cardiotocograph recordings and weekly ultrasound scan of the fetus. Deliver at 37 weeks or if fetal compromise becomes evident.

Before 34 weeks of gestation

In the absence of contraindications such as infection give 2 doses of 12 mg dexamethasone at 12-hourly intervals. Dexamethasone can cause a transient rise in white cell count for 24–36 hours. Before 26 weeks the fetal heart rate change is difficult to interpret but fetal tachycardia is a useful guide for infection. Give appropriate antibiotics for pathogens. Deliver if chorioamnionitis is evident. Consider caesarean section if there is fetal risk.

Adopt the same criteria for induction as described above. Vaginal prostaglandin is not contraindicated.

Breech presentation

Contemporary practice advises attempts at external cephalic version when there is no contraindication; if this is unsuccessful deliver by caesarean section. The mother's informed opinion must be considered. There is no evidence to suggest vaginal delivery is not safe when conditions are satisfactory.

Twin pregnancies

In the absence of obstetric complication induction of labour by amniotomy or use of prostaglandin is not contraindicated. Requirements for twin delivery must be satisfied. Both fetuses should be in cephalic presentation since increasingly breech presentations indicate need for delivery by caesarean section.

Intrauterine fetal death (IUFD)

The main risk with intrauterine fetal death is infection and if the dead fetus is retained more than 4 weeks coagulopathy may develop.

Procedure

- Confirm fetal death by ultrasound scan.
- Support expected expression of grief. Consult with all involved to arrange a mutually acceptable time for induction of labour. Immediate induction of labour after confirmation of intrauterine death need not be the most helpful psychological approach. Onset of coagulopathy can vary. Check platelet count and perform thrombophilic screen.
- Where cervical status is favourable (high Bishop's score) rupture membranes and administer intravenous syntocinon.
- With a low Bishop's score administer prostaglandins as described above. Recently misoprostol, a cost effective option, is also used.
- In very early pregnancies (before 24 weeks of gestation) extra amniotic prostaglandin delivered by placement of a size 12–14 Foley's catheter through the cervix is an option. The balloon is inflated with 20–40 ml of saline to keep the catheter in place. An infusion pump is used to deliver PGE_2 10 mg per ml at a rate of 0.5 ml per hour. This can be increased by 0.5 ml hourly to a maximum dose of 3.0 ml per hour. Augment with syntocinon if delivery is not achieved within 24 hours. Misoprostol followed by misoprostol after 24–36 hours is the current alternative. Cervical laceration and uterine rupture are recognized complications. Examine mother carefully and observe closely for 6 hours after delivery.
- When induction of labour is contraindicated or carries substantial risk, deliver by hysterotomy or caesarean section.

KEY POINTS IN INDUCTION OF LABOUR

- Make sure the mother and her partner are aware of and accept the reasons for and process and risk of induction.

- Decision and assessment for induction of labour must be made by an experienced obstetrician.
- Deliver by caesarean section instead of induction for severe maternal or fetal compromise.
- Deliver by caesarean section when induction for maternal and fetal compromise is unsuccessful.
- Oxytocin by intravenous infusion allows good control of uterine activity. Use the minimum dose which provides adequate uterine contractions.
- The pharmacological effect of oxytocin is potentiated after administration of prostaglandin.
- Once membranes are ruptured aim to deliver within 24 hours to reduce risk of intrauterine infection.
- Close maternal and fetal surveillance is mandatory.

AUGMENTATION OF LABOUR

This process describes enhancement of uterine contractions when progress of labour is slow. Before augmentation exclude malpresentation, gross disproportion and fetal or maternal compromise.

Key points

- Decision to augment labour must follow assessment of situation by experienced obstetrician. This decision must be acceptable to the mother.
- Aim to achieve adequate contractions (frequency of 4–5 contractions per 10 minutes, each contraction lasting 40–60 seconds). Contractions should produce cervical dilatation and descent of the presenting part.
- A wide range of uterine activity can produce cervical dilatation averaging 1 cm per hour.
- Augmentation, like induction of labour, must be conducted with due care. This care includes nursing support, pain relief and close surveillance.

Augmentation before 3 cm cervical dilatation

In the latent phase of labour augmentation is advised after 8 hours of painful contractions occurring at a frequency of 2 every 10 minutes. (WHO 1994). Exclude contraindications to labour.

Augmentation after 3 cm cervical dilatation

This is considered when cervical dilatation drifts 2–3 hours behind the normal partogram (WHO 1994). Exclude contraindications to further labour. Rupture fetal membranes if these are still intact. The same syntocinon regimen as for induction of labour is used. Labour progress is measured in terms of both cervical dilatation and descent of the fetal head. Cervical dilatation without descent of the fetal head forewarns of possible disproportion. Descent of the fetal head without cervical dilatation is associated with cervical fibrosis, for example after cone biopsy.

Close surveillance is mandatory. If fetal compromise develops or little change is detected after 4 hours of adequate contractions deliver by caesarean section.

Obstructed labour in primigravidae leads to incoordinate labour or cessation of uterine activity. In multigravidae the uterus attempts to overcome the obstruction by increasing frequency and intensity of contractions with resultant tetanic uterine activity and risk of uterine rupture.

REFERENCES

World Health Organization Maternal Health and Safe Motherhood programme 1994 World Health Organization partograph in management of labour. Lancet 343: 1399–1404

FURTHER READING

Arulkumaran S, Koh C H, Ingemarsson I, Ratnam S S 1987 Augmentation of labour. Mode of delivery related to cervimetric progress. Australian and New Zealand Journal of Obstetrics and Gynaecology 27: 304–308

Bakketeig L S, Bergsjo P 1989 Post-term pregnancy: magnitude of problem. In: Chalmers I, Enkin M, Keirse M (eds) Effective care in pregnancy and childbirth 765–75. Oxford University Press, London

Bishop E H 1964 Pelvic scoring for elective induction. Obstetrics and Gynecology 24: 266–268

Bouvain M, Iron O 2001 Sweeping the membranes for inducing labour or preventing post-term pregnancy (Cochrane Review). In: The Cochrane Library, Issue 1, 200, Update Software, Oxford

Calder A A 1979 Management of unripe cervix. In: Keirse M N J C, Anderson A B M (eds) Human Parturition. Leiden University Press, Leiden, p 201–217

CESDI 1995 Confidential enquiry into UK stillbirth and neonatal death, 5th annual report. Maternal and Child Health Consortium, London

Crowley P 1995 Elective induction of labour at 41 weeks' gestation. In: Enkin M W, Keirse M J B C, Renfrew M J et al (eds) Pregnancy and children module. The Cochrane Database (disk and CD ROM). The Cochrane Collaboration, Issue 2, Update Software, Oxford

Frait G, Daniel Y, Lessing J B et al 1998 Can labour with breech presentation be induced? Gynecology and Obstetric Investigation 46: 181–186

Friedman E A 1954 The graphic analysis of labour. American Journal of Obstetrics and Gynecology 68: 1569

Johnson T A, Greer I A, Kelly R W, Calder A A 1992 The effect of pH on release of PGE_2 from vaginal and endocervical preparations for induction of labour: an invitro study. British Journal of Obstetrics and Gynaecology 99: 877–880

Liu D T Y, Kerr-Wilson R 1977 Cervical dilatation in spontaneous and induced labours. British Journal of Clinical Practice 31: 177

MacKenzie I Z 1991 Prostaglandin induction and the scarred uterus. Second European Congress on prostaglandins in reproduction, The Hague, Amsterdam. Excerta Medica 29–39

MacKenzie I Z, Magill P, Burns E 1997 Randomised trial of one versus two doses of prostaglandins for induction of labour. I Clinical outcome, II Analysis of cost. British Journal of Obstetrics and Gynaecology 104: 1062–1067

Nuutila M, Kajanoja P 1996 Local administration of prostaglandin E_2 for cervical ripening and labour induction: the appropriate route and dose. Acta Obstetrica Gynecologica Scandinavica 75: 135–138

Royal College of Obstetricians and Gynaecologists 1998 Guidelines on induction of labour. RCOG, London

Tarnow-Mordi W, Shaw J C L, Liu D T Y et al 1981 Iatrogenic hyponatraemia of the newborn due to maternal fluid overload: a prospective study. British Medical Journal 283: 639

Wing D A, Rahall A, Jones M M et al 1995 Misoprostol: an effective agent for cervical ripening and labour induction. American Journal of Obstetrics and Gynecology 172: 1811–1816

16

Assisted vaginal delivery and complications

D. Liu, G. S. H. Yeo

INDICATIONS FOR INSTRUMENTAL ASSISTED VAGINAL DELIVERIES

The incidence of instrumental vaginal delivery should be between 8 and 10% of births.

Maternal indications

- Maternal exhaustion.
- To avoid excessive voluntary expulsive effort where increase in intra-abdominal, intrathoracic and intracranial pressure is best avoided (e.g. maternal cardiac disease, poor respiratory reserves or neurological disorders).

Fetal indications

- Developing fetal compromise when there is good reserve and little calculated difficulty for assisted delivery.
- For the aftercoming head of the breech (by controlled delivery with forceps).

Labour indications

- Malposition (e.g. occipitoposterior and occipitotransverse).
- Prolonged second stage of labour.
- To expedite delivery.

REQUIREMENTS FOR ASSISTED DELIVERY

- There should be a thorough assessment of the forces of the second stage of labour, in particular presence of dystocia, and of the degree of difficulty of the assisted delivery.

- With regard to the fetus, membranes are ruptured, the head is engaged (determined by abdominal palpation and vaginal examination), position of the fetal head is defined and the station is at or below the ischial spines. Fetal ears can be palpated to provide guidance for position of fetal head.
- The mother's cervix is fully dilated. There is adequate anaesthesia. Absolute disproportion is excluded.
- There should be adequate communication between the mother, her partner and medical carers.
- The obstetrician is experienced or supervised by an experienced senior. There must be willingness to abandon the attempt if assisted delivery does not proceed easily.

FACTORS OPERATING IN THE SECOND STAGE OF LABOUR

Successful outcome for assisted delivery is governed by a dynamic balance between the passage, passenger and powers.

Passage and passenger

An accurate assessment of the passage and passenger begins with antenatal care and continues into the intrapartum period.

In the antenatal period, the fetus (or passenger) is continuously monitored for signs of intrauterine growth restriction (IUGR) or macrosomia. Fetal size, presentation, position, attitude and growth are assessed by a combination of abdominal and ultrasound examinations.

The passage is assessed by clinical examination and magnetic resonance and radiological pelvimetry. Gross pelvic contracture can be detected but usefulness of pelvimetry for predicting dystocia is questioned.

Past obstetric history detailing modes of delivery for various birthweights allows estimation of fetal size against past performances to indicate likelihood of dystocia in the current pregnancy.

Gross cephalo–pelvic disproportion must be excluded before any attempt at assisted vaginal delivery. Minor degrees of disproportion are difficult to detect. Possible reduced pelvic diameter and/or a moderately big fetus forewarn likely borderline cephalo–pelvic disproportion and need for assistance.

Powers

Both abdominal palpation and tocographic monitoring detect frequency and duration of uterine contractions but not their intensity. Use of intrauterine pressure catheters for intensity of uterine contractions is not helpful in the management of dystocia.

The forces in the second stage for delivery are:

- uterine contractions
- maternal expulsive effort
- fundal pressure.

Uterine contractions

Uterine contractions will facilitate assisted delivery.

Maternal expulsive effort

Poor maternal effort is a common indication for assisted deliveries. Pushing is both exhausting and ineffective when it is not synchronized with uterine contractions. Advise mother to push to coincide with uterine contractions. Rest between contractions to avoid tiring the mother.

Fundal pressure

Fundal pressure (Fig. 16.1) is used during caesarean births and assisted deliveries. Pressure is applied at the uterine fundus (usually over the buttocks of the fetus) along its longitudinal axis to coincide with uterine contractions and maternal expulsive efforts. Fundal pressure should not be applied in between contractions particularly when maternal effort is absent.

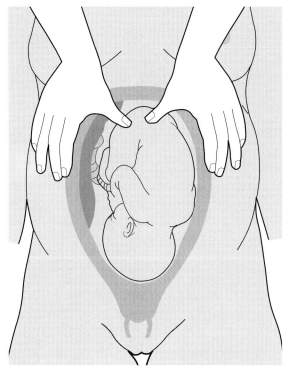

Figure 16.1 Application of fundal pressure: both hands are placed on the fundus of the uterus and a gentle push is applied during contraction.

ASSISTED DELIVERY

Assistance should be in synchrony with expulsive forces to overcome soft tissue resistance in the second stage of labour, usually for delivery of the fetal head. Resistance arises from individual differences in pelvic musculofacial soft tissue, perineal tissue compliance and to some degree moulding of the fetal head.

Informed consent

Assisted vaginal delivery is an operative procedure with its attendant risks and complications hence requires detailed discussion with the mother and her partner. Consent, usually verbal, is often obtained just before an emergency procedure from a distressed mother. Although necessarily brief, discussion and counselling are essential. A more detailed discussion should follow to debrief and answer questions.

Instruments for assisted delivery

Forceps

There are two types of forceps:

1. Traction forceps
   a. with long handles, e.g. Neville Barnes forceps
   b. with short handles for outlet procedures or during caesarean section, e.g. Wrigley's forceps.
2. Rotational forceps, e.g. Kjelland's forceps.

   Description of forceps Each forceps has a left and right fenestrated blade. Each traction blade has a cephalic curve for the fetal head and a pelvic curve to accommodate the curvature of the maternal pelvis. When joined as a pair through a fixed lock, these blades form a protective cage which surrounds the fetal head without compression. When traction is applied, pressure transmitted to the fetus is safely contained by the firm fetal malar bones (Figs 16.2, 16.3).

The Kjelland's rotational forceps differs from traction forceps. The shank is long and the blade is thin. The modest pelvic curve allows rotation through a much smaller circumference. The sliding lock allows application when asynclitism is present (see Ch. 19). Knobs on the handles (also known as occipital knobs) point towards the occiput (Figs 16.4, 16.5 and 16.6).

Vacuum extractors

Vacuum extractors can have rigid cups or soft cups. Rigid cups in use are:

- Malmstrom – anterior cup
- Bird – anterior and posterior cup
- O'Neill – anterior and posterior cup
- Mityvac – anterior cup
- Kiwi Omnicup – universal anterior and posterior cup.

Soft cups in use are:

- Silc cup – anterior cup
- Silastic cup – anterior cup.

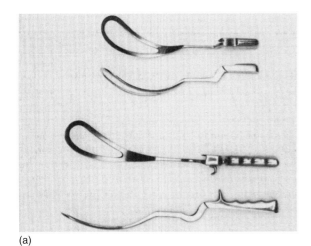

(a)

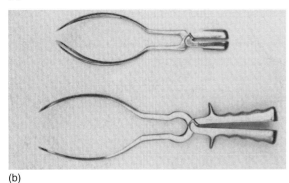

(b)

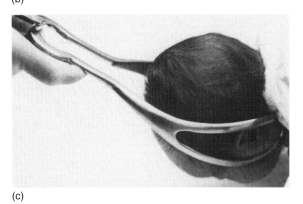

(c)

Figure 16.2 Large and small traction forceps (a) as separates, (b) as pairs and (c) applied.

Description of vacuum extractor The principal components of the vacuum extractor are the pump, the pressure gauge, the traction piece and the cup used to raise the chignon for traction (Fig. 16.7). Figure 16.8 shows a modern Ventouse extractor and delivery system.

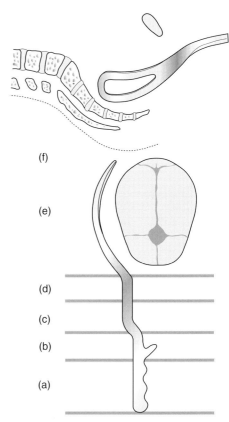

(f)

(e)

(d)

(c)

(b)

(a)

Figure 16.3 Traction forceps illustrating (a) handle, (b) shoulder, (c) lock, (d) shank, (e) blade with cephalic curve and (f) pelvic curve.

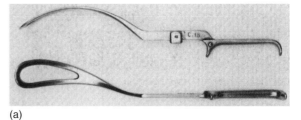

(a)

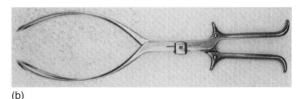

(b)

Figure 16.4 Kjelland's forceps (a) as separates and (b) paired.

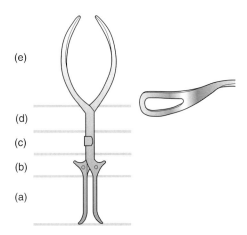

Figure 16.5 Components of Kjelland's forceps: (a) handle, (b) shoulder, (c) sliding lock, (d) shank and (e) blade.

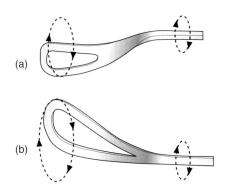

Figure 16.6 Rotation of Kjelland's forceps (b) is through a smaller circumference than with the traction forceps (a).

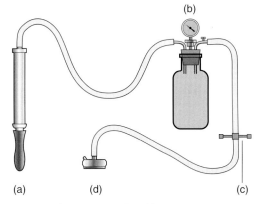

Figure 16.7 Components of the Ventouse extractor: (a) pump, (b) container with pressure gauge, (c) traction piece and (d) cup.

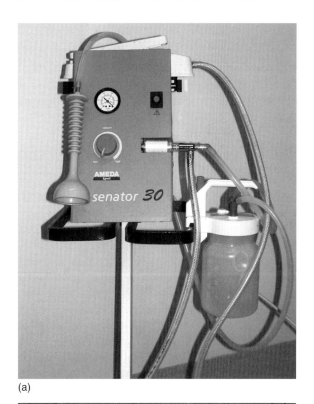

(a)

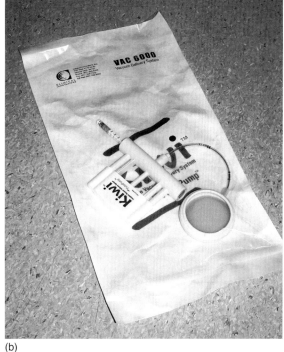

(b)

Figure 16.8 (a) Contemporary Ventouse extractor. (b) Vacuum delivery system.

Choice between forceps or vacuum extraction for assisted deliveries

Contemporary reviews show that vacuum extraction compared to forceps delivery is associated with significantly less maternal trauma (Chalmers & Chalmers 1989, Drife 1996, Johanson & Menon 1999, Meniru 1996). Fewer caesarean sections were carried out in the vacuum extractor group. However, the vacuum extractor was associated with an increase in neonatal cephalohaematoma and retinal haemorrhages. Forceps are associated with a lower failure rate. The chief disadvantage of forceps delivery is a higher risk of significant maternal perineal injury.

Neither instrument is superior for assisted vaginal deliveries. The forces and requirements for both forms of assisted deliveries are similar. The instrument of choice depends on the clinical scenario as well as the operator's experience, training and preferences. Both instruments are equally suited in most assisted deliveries. In circumstances where cephalopelvic disproportion is confidently excluded and speed is of essence (e.g. ominous cardiotocographic tracing), the forceps can be the instrument of choice for expediting delivery. The vacuum extractor may be preferred where asynclitism is present, when rotational delivery is needed and when there is limited experience with forceps. There is no increased morbidity in completing a delivery by forceps when the vacuum failed, provided that the requirements for assisted delivery are fulfilled (see above). Table 16.1 shows a comparison between the two types of instrumental vaginal delivery.

TRACTION PROCEDURES

Box 16.1 describes types of traction procedures used in assisted delivery.

Before application of instruments

- Indications and requirements – ensure that these have been met.
- Communication with colleagues – inform consultant (if appropriate), anaesthetist and

Table 16.1 Instrumental vaginal delivery

Conditions	Forceps	Vacuum
Popularity	Decreased	Increased
Preterm	Yes	Not before 36 weeks
Undilated cervix (around 9 cm)	Contraindicated	Yes
Anaesthesia	Yes	Need less
Failure to achieve delivery	Less likely	More likely
Tissue trauma	Possible	Less
Cephalohaematoma	Possible	More likely
Retinal haemorrhage	Possible	More likely
Postpartum perineal pain	Yes	Less

Box 16.1 Traction procedures used in assisted delivery

- Outlet procedure describes the situation where the scalp is visible and the fetal head is at or on the perineum.
- Low procedure is when the fetal skull is at station +2 or more.
- Mid-pelvic procedure refers to the situation where the head is engaged but the station is between 0 and +2.

---

operating theatre staff (if a trial of forceps in operating theatre is indicated), and neonatologist (especially if the indication is for fetal distress).

- Informed consent – obtain verbal consent after explaining to mother and her partner the need for assisted delivery. Warn the mother that intense pressure and the sensation of pelvic separation may be felt at the moment of birth. This is the normal experience of childbirth. Unless forewarned, especially in a nulliparous mother, this frightening sensation could be wrongly attributed to the misuse of instruments or obstetric ineptitude.
- Position – the lithotomy position is favoured. The legs are suspended by stirrups or other means. Adopt a 15° left lateral tilt to overcome supine hypotension.
- Bladder – empty the bladder to avoid damage during traction and/or rotation.

During the use of instruments

1. Position of the obstetrician – the flexed forearm is at the level of the vulva or slightly lower (Fig. 16.9).

2. Position of the mother – the perineum should slightly overhang the edge of the bed. There should be room below the buttock for assisted deliveries, especially for rotational forceps.

3. Check the instrument. For forceps delivery check that both blades lock easily and are well lubricated. For vacuum assisted delivery: check that the traction chain and the tubings are airtight; check that the suction apparatus and the vacuum have been connected properly; choose the appropriate cup size (the largest cup possible should be used).

4. Reassure mother and partner. Discourage pushing during insertion of the blades. The partner's prime role is support and not as a spectator.

5. Apply the instrument as described in Box 16.2.

6. Check application. For forceps:
   a. Ensure that the sagittal suture is in the midline, equidistant between the blades (Fig. 16.10).

b. The posterior fontanelle should be one finger's breadth above the shanks (for OA position).
   c. The fenestrated blades should admit one finger between the heel of the blade and the fetal head.

For vacuum:
   a. Ensure that the centre of the cup is over the sagittal suture and 3 cm anterior to the posterior fontanelle.
   b. Check that the mother's cervical and vaginal mucosa have been excluded from the cup before traction.

7. Apply gentle traction. The vacuum cup is held against the fetal head with the thumb and index finger of the left hand to detect any tendency of the cup to separate. Check repeatedly with index finger to detect inclusion of cervix and vagina into the vacuum.
   a. Apply traction during uterine contractions and bearing down efforts – in line with the pelvic axis (Fig. 16.14). Pajot's manoeuvre may be used with the forceps. Traction is applied perpendicular to the cup in the direction of the pelvic axis when the vacuum is used (Fig. 16.15).

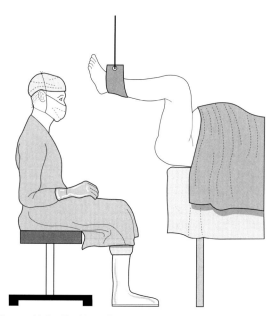

Figure 16.9 Position of an obstetrician for forceps delivery. Mother's legs are suspended by stirrups or other means.

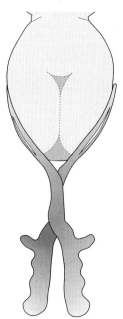

Figure 16.10 Position of sagittal suture with correct application of forceps.

Box 16.2 Application of instruments

Forceps

1. Insert the left blade first.
   a. Check that there is no uterine contraction and that the mother is not pushing.
   b. Place the index and middle fingers of the right hand along the left side of the fetal head to exclude the vaginal walls (Fig. 16.11).
   c. The left hand holds the blade vertical and by dropping the handles slips the forceps into position guided by the palmar aspects of the intravaginal fingers.
   d. The blade rests over the fetal ear and malar bones.
2. Repeat the procedure for the right blade.
   a. The right hand now holds the blades which are guided into position by the left index and middle fingers.
   b. The blades should fall together into position.
3. If resistance is felt, check to ensure that all the requirements for forceps delivery are met.
4. Lock the two blades – no undue force should be used. If the blades do not lock easily reassess the situation. The blades are then reapplied.

Vacuum

1. Lubricate the cup.
2. Insert it sideways through the introitus (Fig. 16.12). Aim to position the centre of the cup 3 cm anterior to the posterior fontanelle and over the sagittal suture. This will maintain the head in the optimal maximum flex attitude. Avoid placement over fontanelle.
3. Exclude cervix and folds of vaginal mucosa.

4. Create an initial vacuum up to 0.2 kPa over 1–2 minutes. Check again that cervix and vaginal mucosa have been excluded from the cup.
5. The vacuum pressure is raised to a working pressure of 0.8 kPa.
6. Once working pressure is achieved wait for 30 seconds for the chignon to form before applying traction (Fig. 16.13).

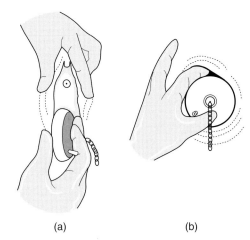

(a)   (b)

Figure 16.12 (a) Insertion and (b) application of cups.

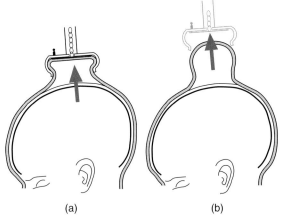

(a)   (b)

Figure 16.13 (a) Formation of a chignon to assist traction (b) with residue swelling persisting for 24–48 hours after cup is removed.

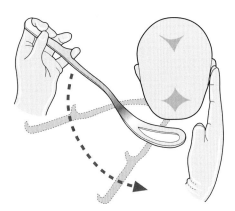

Figure 16.11 Application of traction forceps.

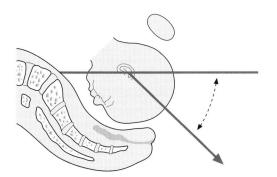

Figure 16.14 Traction in line with pelvic axis.

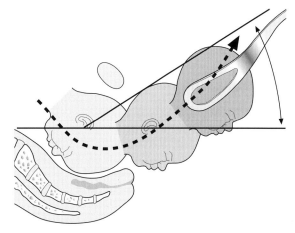

Figure 16.16 Delivery of head with forceps.

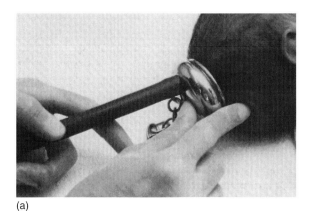

(a)

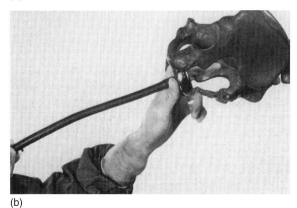

(b)

Figure 16.15 (a) Placement of intravaginal fingers and (b) direction of traction.

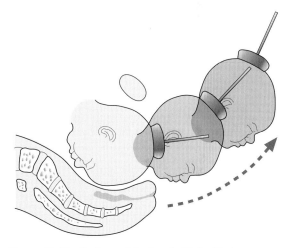

Figure 16.17 Delivery of the head with the Ventouse extractor.

b. No more than 15–20 kg of pull is required to achieve delivery.

c. Apply traction for 20–30 seconds at a time. Delivery should be achieved with 3 or fewer pulls (Fig. 16.16). More than 30 minutes of vacuum can result in scalp necrosis.

d. An episiotomy is usually required as the vertex is crowning.

e. Change direction of traction to 30° from the horizontal once the vertex (chin in face presentation) emerges beneath the symphysis (Fig. 16.17). Failure to change direction is an important cause of trauma to the perineum.

f. After crowning ask mother to stop pushing and start panting. Panting will produce gentle intermittent intra-abdominal pressure which nudges the baby slowly out of the birth canal.

Delivery of the baby

- Deliver the head slowly to avoid tears to the perineum or extension of the episiotomy.
- Once the head is delivered, the blades of the forceps are disengaged (or the vacuum is released and the cup removed).
- The rest of the delivery is the same as that for normal birth.

Procedures after delivery

- Check arterial and venous cord pH and base excess.
- Examine the pelvic structures to exclude damage. Locate the apex of the episiotomy to check for extension. Rotational deliveries are more likely to cause damage.
- Jointly with the neonatologist conduct examination of the baby (including any soft tissue injuries). Communicate findings of the baby to the parents and reassure if appropriate.
- Document fully findings, discussions with mother and her partner, steps of the procedure and condition of the mother and baby after delivery (including Apgar score and cord pH).

ROTATIONAL PROCEDURES

A wider diameter is presented when the vertex is in the occipitolateral or occipitoposterior position. Rotation into the anteroposterior diameter of the pelvic outlet may occur on the perineum or at any level between the ischial spines and the perineum. Delivery in the occipitoposterior position may increase perineal trauma unless carefully conducted.

The three most common techniques used for placing the vertex into the anteroposterior diameter of the pelvic outlet are:

- Rotation by hand (manual)
- Rotation with a vacuum extractor
- Rotation with Kjelland's forceps.

Requirements

- Include requirements for assisted vaginal deliveries. Ensure adequate anaesthesia at level of rotation.
- A neonatologist should be in attendance.
- If any difficulty is anticipated, the procedure should be conducted in the operating theatre with provisions made for immediate caesarean section.

Manual rotation

This is a safe technique. Pressure on the fetal head is easy to judge and trauma to soft tissue is less likely. Check cervical dilatation and adequacy of pelvis.

Technique

- Confirm the malposition.
- Lubricate the traction forceps and place them within reach.
- The left hand is used for right occipitolateral or posterior positions, the right hand is used for left occipitolateral or posterior positions.
- Insert the hand into the vagina to grasp the fetal head across the parietal diameter with thumb uppermost. Use thumb, index and middle finger if access is limited (Fig. 16.18).
- Disimpact the fetal head and rotate the occiput anteriorly. Place the free hand over the mother's

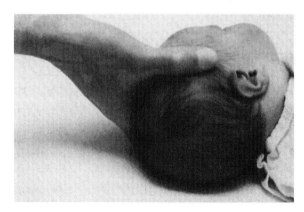

Figure 16.18 Position of hand for manual rotation.

abdomen in the region of the anterior fetal shoulder. The shoulder is brought across the midline towards the opposite iliac crest to assist rotation at the same time as rotation of the vertex. An assistant can help prevent tendency of the shoulder to revert to its original position. Flexion with contraction is often evident with correct rotation.

- Whilst the vertex is held in the occipitoanterior position, the forceps blades are applied in the usual manner. Check correct alignment of the sagittal suture.
- Difficulties in locking the blades suggest inadequate rotation and hence incorrect application of the forceps.
- Apply traction only after application of the forceps is judged to be correct.

Ventouse rotation

Technique

- Apply the cup well back on the fetal head so that traction corrects any deflexion which is usual in malposition.
- Asynclitism (see Ch. 19) is almost always present in malposition and is corrected by a more posterior application of the cup.
- Initial traction down towards the floor allows the vertex to descend and correct asynclitism. Rotation usually takes place at the pelvic floor level. The thumb and index finger in the vagina to ensure contact between cup and the scalp can also help rotation by directing cup in direction of turn.
- After successful rotation, complete the delivery by maintaining traction perpendicular to the cup in line with the pelvic axis.

Rotation by Kjelland's forceps

In these forceps designed for rotation the shank is long and the blade thin. There is no pelvic curve so rotation is through a smaller circumference. The sliding locks allow application when asynclitism is present.

Application by wandering anterior blade

- Check placement of the blades by assembling them in front of the pelvis. Ensure that the directional knobs point towards the occiput.
- Select the anterior blade (the blade which will be placed on the upper surface of the fetal head). The second and third fingers of the hand on the side of the fetal face are inserted into the vagina (Fig. 16.19).
- The anterior blade, held vertically by the free hand, is slipped into the vagina between the fetal face and the intravaginal fingers. The handle is depressed towards the floor at the same time. The face is chosen because the bitemporal diameter, being smaller than the biparietal diameter, provides for easier application.
- When the blade is two-thirds of the way inside the vagina, the handle is nearly horizontal. The handle is rotated towards the floor from this position whilst the intravaginal fingers assist the passage of the blade across the fetal face. When the blade is positioned correctly over the ear and malar bone the handle is raised so that the blade will encompass the full length of the fetal head (Fig. 16.20).
- Sometimes the occiput rotates into the direct occipitoposterior position during the application of the wandering blade. The Kjelland's forceps can then be inserted directly with the knobs pointing towards the occiput.

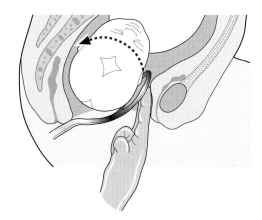

Figure 16.19   Application of anterior blade.

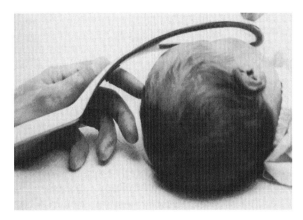

Figure 16.20 Direction of blade over fetal face by intravaginal digits.

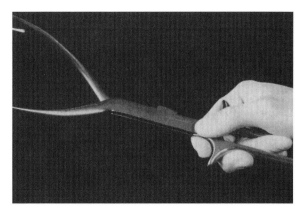

Figure 16.21 Grip technique for rotation.

- If difficulty is encountered withdrawing the blade a short distance can help. Alternatively apply blade across occiput.

Application by the direct method

- The anterior blade is held vertically with the handle pointing towards the floor. The cephalic curve is placed in contact with the fetal head at the level of the ears and malar bones. Two intravaginal fingers guide placement of the blade as the handle is elevated.
- The posterior blade is always applied directly to the head. Intravaginal fingers guide the blade into position. The tip of the blade is always kept close to the fetal head. When applied correctly there should be no difficulty in locking the blades. Presence of asynclitism would mean that the shoulders of the handles are not at the same level.

Rotation and delivery

- When correctly applied, the handles are at 45° from the horizontal and in line with the pelvic axis. Vertical direction of the handles greater than 45° indicates that the head is not fully engaged and it may be safer to abandon the procedure.
- Correct asynclitism by adjusting the handles so that the shoulders of the blades are level. Sometimes this is easier during a contraction.

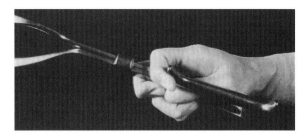

Figure 16.22 Grip technique for traction.

- The blades are held by the shoulders. The fourth finger is interposed between the handles to remind the obstetrician not to compress them. This particular grip for rotation prevents excessive force being used and is highly sensitive to the presence of unnecessary resistance (Fig. 16.21).
- The fetal head is rotated at the level of application of the forceps. The rotational force needed is usually not more than what is comfortably applied with two fingers. If difficulty is encountered, rotation may be achieved with descent during the next contraction. Occasionally moving fetal head up a few centimetres allows rotation at the widest pelvic plane.
- Once rotation is achieved, the grip is changed to facilitate traction (Fig. 16.22). Traction must be along the pelvic axis (Fig. 16.23). Interpose thumb between handles. Pajot's manoeuvre can help (Fig. 16.24).

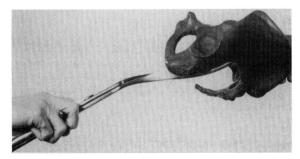

Figure 16.23 Axis traction.

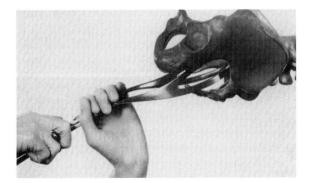

Figure 16.24 Axis traction with Pajot's manoeuvre to maintain traction in pelvic axis.

- An episiotomy is made in the usual manner. Do not make an episiotomy before rotation otherwise the spiral torque during rotation may cause extension of the episiotomy.

Inherent dangers of Kjelland's forceps

There are two inherent dangers in the design of the Kjelland's forceps. Firstly, the thin blades can cause considerable soft tissue trauma. Secondly, the wandering technique necessitates moving the blades over a large area of vagina. This increases the risk of trauma. Whether Kjelland's forceps should continue to be used is controversial.

TRIAL OF FORCEPS OR VACUUM

- All potentially difficult forceps or vacuum deliveries should be conducted as a trial by an experienced obstetrician.
- The trial should be conducted in the operating theatre with immediate access to caesarean

section if the trial fails (remember prophylactic citrates, informed consent, intravenous line and grouped blood available at short notice). The neonatologist, anaesthetist and theatre staff must be in attendance. Do not perform episiotomy until vaginal delivery is assured.

- The trial fails when there is no advance or little descent with a moderate amount of traction. A trial of forceps after use of vacuum should only be performed if the operator is confident vaginal delivery is possible and the fetal head is deeply engaged. Only then is delivery accomplished without harm to the mother or baby. Note reason for failure with the first instrument. Check requirements for assisted deliveries are met.
- Leave an indwelling catheter, disimpact the fetal head and place it above the level of ischial spines to facilitate delivery of the head by caesarean section when trial of vaginal delivery fails.

MATERNAL COMPLICATIONS

Assisted vaginal deliveries are associated with the following complications:

- Perineal and vaginal lacerations, extension of episiotomy, third degree tears and haematoma formation. A thorough examination must be performed after delivery is achieved. Injury to the urethral–vesical angle and anal sphincter can lead to immediate problems such as difficulty with voiding or subsequent urinary and faecal incontinence.
- Vaginal haematoma formation and laceration can occur with spontaneous vaginal deliveries but are more likely after rotational instrument delivery. Severe laceration, particularly if the vaginal vault is involved, may require laparotomy and extended surgery, hence an experienced obstetrician must be present. Haematomas following rupture of vaginal veins will need evacuation if large, painful or judged to be enlarging.
- Do not perform instrumental delivery unless the cervix is fully dilated. Exceptions include vacuum delivery for the second twin or need

for urgent vaginal delivery at 9 cm cervical dilatation when requirements for easy delivery are met. Torn cervix leading to maternal death has been reported with use of the vacuum. Again experience is mandatory before attempt at repair of cervical lacerations especially if there is extension into the fornix. Minor lacerations that are not bleeding can be managed expectantly.

- The lumbosacral nerves may be impinged upon by movement of the sacroiliac joints, compression by the fetal presenting part or use of forceps. Transient loss of sensory and motor function may result.

NEONATAL COMPLICATIONS

- Risk of perinatal trauma in instrumental vaginal delivery correlates with duration of attempt, level of the fetal head in the birth canal, need for rotation and condition of baby at start of procedure.
- Compared to forceps, the vacuum is associated with higher rates of neonatal trauma. These include cephalohaematoma with neonatal hyperbilirubinaemia needing phototherapy, scalp injuries and retinal haemorrhage.
- Chignon or swelling of the scalp which develops when vacuum is applied is observed when the cup is removed. This swelling, which becomes diffused within an hour to behave like a normal caput succedaneum, usually disappears over 1 or 2 days. Scalp markings or abrasions can last as long as 6 months after delivery.
- Subcutaneous haematomas resolve in a few days. Cephalohaematomas may take up to a few weeks to disappear. Reassure parents.
- Neonatal jaundice is more common after vacuum extraction than after forceps or spontaneous delivery. There is no difference in the number of babies requiring phototherapy.
- Subgaleal haemorrhage associated with difficult instrumental delivery is more likely when fetal hypoxia or coagulopathy is present. This life-threatening condition is a serious complication associated with vacuum extraction. Intracranial

haemorrhage can also complicate difficult vacuum extractions.
- Retinal haemorrhage, more common after instrumental delivery than after normal birth, is significantly more likely after vacuum extraction than after forceps delivery. This is a transient lesion.

MEDICAL LEGAL ISSUES

Instrumental vaginal delivery followed by complications or poor fetal outcome is a ready situation for complaints and litigation. The following are important from a clinical governance and risk management perspective:

- Appropriate assessment of the situation is vital. Obstetric history, presence of maternal or fetal compromise, good appreciation of pelvic diameters and configurations, mother's preference, available expertise and option for caesarean section are all important issues.
- The obstetrician must be adequately trained or supervised.
- The mother and partner must be made aware of need, likely outcome and options. Obtain consent and maintain communication to inform and reassure.
- There is no place for instrumental delivery if the obstetrician cannot properly assess the pelvis and relate fetal head size to pelvic diameters and outlet.
- Be prepared to abandon procedure when difficulty is encountered and when there is little descent with traction. Avoid repeated attempts and use of multiple instruments. Forceps can be considered after failure with the vacuum. The reverse sequence is not acceptable.
- Detailed documentation is essential. This includes indication, discussion with mother and partner regarding risks and options, any complication and remedial action, condition of mother and baby, cord arterial and venous values.
- Full explanation and prompt attention to complications are important. Offer apology where appropriate.

- Introduce audit for individual obstetrician and the labour ward as a whole to ensure continuous quality control.

SYMPHYSIOTOMY

This procedure is seldom used but can be effective for delivery if the aftercoming head of a normal live breech is stuck at the pelvic outlet.

Procedure

- Lithotomy position.
- General, regional or local anaesthesia.
- Catheterized bladder. Leave catheter indwelling.
- Incise skin above symphysis with firm blade. Probe with blade to identify non bony joint.
- Displace urethra from midline by a finger in the vagina.
- Hold blade at 30° from horizontal and advance vertically down towards the vagina. Use a sawing action till the tip of the blade is sensed by the intra-vaginal finger.
- Once the joint separates apply forceps and deliver the fetal head. An episiotomy is helpful.

Precautions

- Avoid wide separation of symphysis to protect sacroiliac joint and urethra.
- Insert drain if there is venous bleeding when arcuate ligaments are cut.
- Leave catheter in situ for 48 hours.
- Support pelvic girdle and nurse mother on her side.

SHOULDER DYSTOCIA

This term describes difficulty with delivery of the shoulder after delivery of the fetal head. This unpredictable emergency occurs in 0.5–2% of vaginal deliveries. The complication is usually due to the anterior shoulder becoming stuck above the symphysis pubis.

Risk factors include:

- Fetal macrosomia. Incidence increases from 10 to 20% for birthweight between 4250 g and 4750 g.

- Diabetic mothers. Risk compared to non-diabetics is increased by more than 70% for similar birthweight.
- Prolonged labour and long second stage (70% are associated with normal labours).
- Past history of shoulder dystocia (over 50% incidence of shoulder dystocias are in babies weighing less than 4000 g).

Management

Antenatal

- Neither clinical nor ultrasound diagnosis of macrosomia is reliable.
- There is no evidence that induction at full term is helpful but benefit of earlier delivery at 37–38 weeks remains a subject for investigation.
- There is a place for elective caesarean section when estimated fetal weight is more than 4500 g, when likely macrosomia accompanies diabetes and for a definite history of previous difficulty with shoulder dystocia.
- Forewarn at-risk mothers to ensure their delivery is in hospital. Document clearly to alert labour ward staff.

Intrapartum

All labour ward medical staff must be regularly drilled to become practised in managing this emergency.

1. Assess all mothers admitted for delivery. If risk is suspected make sure an experienced obstetrician attends delivery.

2. When this emergency arises activate the following steps:

    a. Recruit help from an experienced midwife, a senior obstetrician, anaesthetist and paediatrician.

    b. Adopt McRoberts' manoeuvre. Flex mother's thighs against abdomen and chest. Offer assistance if she cannot do this herself. The manoeuvre straightens the lumbo–sacral angle and rotates the symphysis superiorly thus opening the pelvic outlet. This manoeuvre alone is effective in resolving 80% of cases of this emergency.

The left lateral position is seldom used. Squatting or knee to chest on all fours position achieves the same advantages but delivery in this position requires experience.

c. Perform an episiotomy to remove soft tissue resistance and allow better access for subsequent steps.

d. Apply suprapubic pressure with flat of hand to free the shoulder, to adduct and reduce the biacromial diameter and direct the shoulder beneath the symphysis into the anteroposterior widest diameter of the pelvic outlet. This step improves delivery rate by an additional 3%.

e. If delivery is not achieved adopt Woods' corkscrew manoeuvre. Insert appropriate hand into posterior vagina and rotate posterior shoulder clockwise or anti-clockwise 180°. This will bring the impacted anterior shoulder below the level of the symphysis to allow delivery.

f. If above steps fail employ Mazzanati procedure to deliver posterior arm. Flex arm at the elbow. The hand or forearm is grasped and swept across the baby's chest and face. The anterior shoulder is disimpacted and slides out beneath the symphysis. The baby's clavicle or humerus may be fractured (18% risk).

g. Impaction of both the anterior shoulder against the symphysis and the posterior shoulder in the sacral promontory necessitate resort to Zavanelli's option. Rotate baby's head into anteroposterior position. Flex the head and push it into the pelvis. Deliver by caesarean section. Maternal morbidity must be considered.

Points to remember

- If one manoeuvre fails move quickly to the next to avoid delay.

- Brachial plexus injury follows excessive or prolonged traction to fetal neck.
- Keep detailed records of all procedures and outcomes.

Post partum

- Enlist neonatologist assistance. Check for presence of injury to baby and mother.
- When appropriate discuss events with mother and her partner to answer questions and agree plans for future pregnancies.

HAEMATOMAS

A shearing action between the vagina and deeper tissues during normal, assisted or rotational delivery can rupture the vaginal plexus of veins to form a haematoma. If extensive, this will involve the paravaginal space, the labia, urethra and even extension into the broad ligament. Inadequate haemostasis following episiotomy repair or closure of caesarean section wound also result in haematoma formation.

Management

- Presents as pain, bruising, urinary retention and, if extensive, hypovolaemic consequences.
- Vaginal examination and, if indicated, ultrasound scan will help diagnosis.
- Small haematomas can be managed conservatively. Catherization is required if the urethra is involved.
- For large haematomas an experienced obstetrician must attend to assess the situation. Surgery, on occasion laparotomy, may be required to evacuate the clots and secure haemostasis. Transfusion may be necessary. Leave drains after surgery if oozing is anticipated.

REFERENCES

Chalmers J A, Chalmers I 1989 The obstetric vacuum extractor is the instrument of first choice for operative vaginal delivery. British Journal of Obstetrics and Gynaecology 96: 505–506

Drife J O 1996 Choice and instrumental delivery. British Journal of Obstetrics and Gynaecology 103: 608–611

Johanson R B, Menon B K V 1999 Vacuum extraction vs forceps delivery (Cochrane Review). In: The Cochrane Library, Issue 4. Update Software, Oxford

Meniru G I 1996 An analysis of recent trends in vacuum extraction and forceps delivery in the United Kingdom. British Journal of Obstetrics and Gynaecology 103: 168–170

FURTHER READING

Acker D B, Sachs B B, Friedman E A 1985 Risk factors for shoulder dystocia. Obstetrics and Gynecology 66: 762–766

Chan C C T, Malathi I, Yeo G S 1999 Is the vacuum extractor really the instrument of first choice? Australia and New Zealand Journal of Obstetrics and Gynaecology 39: 305–309

Drife J O 1996 Choice and instrumental delivery. British Journal of Obstetrics and Gynaecology 103: 608–611

Fortune P M, Thomas R M 1999 Sub-aponeurotic haemorrhage: a rare but life-threatening neonatal complication associated with ventouse delivery. British Journal of Obstetrics and Gynaecology 106: 868–870

Gherman R B, Goodwin T M, Soutar I et al 1997 The McRoberts' manoeuvre for alleviation of shoulder dystocia: how successful is it? American Journal of Obstetrics and Gynaecology 176: 656–661

Gonen R, Spiegel D, Abend M 1996 Is macrosomia predictable, and are shoulder dystocia and birth trauma preventable? Obstetrics and Gynecology 88: 526–529

Gonen O, Rosen D J, Dolfin Z et al 1997 Induction of labour versus expectant management in macrosomia: a randomised study. Obstetrics and Gynecology 89: 913–917

Johanson R B, Heycock E, Carter J et al 1999 Maternal and child health after assisted vaginal delivery: five year follow up of a randomised controlled study comparing forceps and ventouse. British Journal of Obstetrics and Gynaecology 106: 544–549

Johnstone F D, Myerscough P R 1998 Shoulder dystocia. British Journal of Obstetrics and Gynaecology 105: 811–815

Leaphard W L M M C, Capeless E L 1997 Labour induction with a perinatal diagnosis of fetal macrosomia. Journal of Fetal Medicine 6: 99–102

Leather A T 1993 The management of shoulder dystocia. Contemporary Reviews in Obstetrics and Gynaecology 5: 61–64

Louise D F, Raymond R C, Perkins M B et al 1995 Recurrence rate of shoulder dystocia. American Journal of Obstetrics and Gynecology 172: 1369–1371

Luria S, Benarie A, Hugay Z 1994 The ABC of shoulder dystocia management. Asia Oceania Journal of Obstetrics and Gynecology 20: 195–197

Morales R, Adair C D, Sanchez-Ramos L, Gaudier F L 1995 Vacuum extraction of preterm infants with birthweights of 1500–2499 grams. Journal of Reproductive Medicine 40: 127–130

Nesbitt T S, Gilbert W M, Herrchen B 1998 Shoulder dystocia and associated risk factors with macrosomic infants born in California. American Journal of Obstetrics and Gynecology 179: 476–480

Petroikovksy B 1998 Emergency symphysiotomy: too little too late. American Journal of Obstetrics and Gynecology 178: 631–632

Schwartz B C, Dixon D M 1958 Shoulder dystocia. Obstetrics and Gynecology 11: 468–471

Sultan A A, Johanson R B, Carter J E 1998 Occult anal sphincter trauma following randomised forceps and vacuum delivery. International Journal of Obstetrics and Gynaecology 61: 113–119

Towner D, Castro M A, Eby-Wilkens E, Gilbert W M 1999 Effect of mode of delivery in nulliparous women on neonatal intracranial injury. New England Journal of Medicine 341: 1709–1714

Vacca A 1999 The trouble with vacuum extraction. Current Obstetrics Gynaecology 9: 41–45

Vasket T F, Allen A C 1995 Perinatal implication of shoulder dystocia. Obstetrics and Gynecology 86: 142–147

17

Caesarean section

D. Liu, A. Omu

INTRODUCTION

Caesarean section describes the surgical procedure for delivery of the fetus by incisions through the abdomen and uterus. The attendant risk of a surgical procedure must be considered. In the UK the mortality rates for elective procedures stayed between 15 and 17 per 100 000 maternities for 1991–1996 (DoH 1998). Pulmonary embolism, haemorrhage and sepsis continue as salient causes of mortality. Inappropriate delegation, inadequate facilities and poor communication contribute to substandard care and necessitate improvement.

Sequelae of vaginal birth such as rectal and urinary incontinence, the question of choice, increased safety for caesarean section, a greater number of older mothers having babies and ready recourse to litigation for complication with operative vaginal deliveries are factors towards an increase in caesarean section rates.

INDICATIONS FOR CAESAREAN SECTION

Caesarean section can be subdivided into elective, planned emergency, unplanned emergency and peri-mortem and post-mortem categories to facilitate audit. Clearly complications and mortality attributed to the surgical procedure must be distinguished from contributions by the presence of obstetric complications and maternal medical problems.

Caesarean sections are performed:

- to overcome cephalo–pelvic disproportion and abnormal uterine activity

- to expedite delivery for maternal or fetal reasons
- to reduce fetal trauma (e.g. the small preterm breech) and fetal infection (e.g. risk of transmitting herpetic infection or the human immunodeficiency virus)
- to reduce maternal risk (e.g. certain cardiac disorders, intracranial lesions or cervical malignancy)
- to allow mothers to exercise their informed choice.

PREOPERATIVE CARE

- Ensure reason for surgery is valid. There should be input by senior colleagues and clear discussion with mother and her partner.
- Past obstetric and medical history must be reviewed. Check gestation.
- Discuss mode of anaesthesia with the anaesthetist and mother.
- Ideally mode of anaesthesia or analgesia should be discussed in advance at a joint clinic with the anaesthetist.
- Inform the paediatrician in good time.
- Check that cross-matched blood is available. Most labour wards now reserve 2 units of O Rhesus negative blood for emergencies.
- Give an antacid (see Ch. 9).
- Obtain written consent.
- Administer prophylactic antibiotics. This is particularly relevant in emergency caesarean sections. Assess need for prophylaxis against thrombo-embolism. Mothers with three or more moderate risk factors such as age more than 35, obesity of more than 80 kg, para four, gross varicose veins, concurrent infection, pre-eclampsia, 4 days immobility prior to surgery, major medical disease, extended pelvic surgery, personal or family history of venous thrombosis or pulmonary embolism (thrombophilia) and presence of antiphospholipid antibody will need heparin prophylaxis and leg stockings.

POSTOPERATIVE CARE

Presence of obstetric or medical complications means some mothers will need close observation following caesarean section. The labour ward can serve as an area for recovery and care. Intensive or high dependency care facilities must be readily available in the same hospital. General care for all mothers includes:

- Assess vital signs at regular intervals (15 min). Make sure condition is stable.
- Watch fundal height, any bleeding from wound and amount of lochia. This is particularly important if the labour is prolonged, when the uterus has been distended by polyhydramnios or multiple pregnancies and where there is a threat of coagulation defects, for example after antepartum haemorrhage and pre-eclamptic toxaemia.
- Maintain fluid balance.
- Ensure adequate analgesia. Continued use of epidural analgesia is particularly useful.
- Address specific requirements which prompt indication for caesarean section, e.g. medical conditions such as diabetes.
- Encourage early physiotherapy and ambulation if there is no contraindication.
- Remember thrombo-prophylaxis. Early ambulation and attention to hydration suffice for low-risk mothers with uncomplicated pregnancies and no risk factors. Avoid use of Dextran 70. Subcutaneous heparin or mechanical methods are required where risk is considered moderate. Where risk of thrombo-embolism is high, heparin and leg stockings should be used for 5 days following surgery. For past histories of venous thrombo-embolism in pregnancy or the puerperium, thrombo-prophylaxis should be continued for 6 weeks post partum.
- Before discharge an opportunity should be made available to examine events and address questions.
- Schedule an opportunity for postnatal review to ensure complete recovery, to discuss subsequent pregnancies and to ensure follow-up care for medical conditions.

TYPES OF INCISION

Abdominal incisions

Essentially these are the subumbilical midline and transverse lower abdominal incisions (Fig. 17.1).

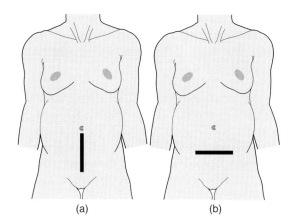

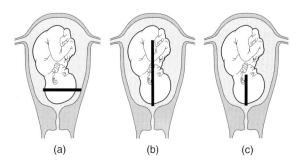

(a)   (b)   (c)

Figure 17.2 Uterine incisions: (a) lower segment, (b) classical and (c) Kronig–Gellhorn–Beck.

(a)   (b)

Figure 17.1 Abdominal incisions: (a) subumbilical midline and (b) transverse 'Pfannenstiel'.

Subumbilical midline incision

This incision is easy and quick. Access is good with minimal bleeding. It is useful when access to the lower segment is difficult, for example in the presence of severe kyphosclerosis or anterior lower segment fibroid. The scar, however, is unsightly, there is more postoperative discomfort and dehiscence is more likely compared with transverse incisions.

Where extension upwards into the abdomen is likely, a left or right paramedian incision can be performed.

Transverse (Pfannenstiel's) incision

This is the current incision of choice. It is cosmetically pleasing, less likely to dehisce and being less uncomfortable allows better post-operative mobility. The incision can be technically more difficult especially in repeat surgery. It can be more vascular and provides less access.

Variations include the Joel Cohen incision (place higher up the abdomen) and Misgav Ladach (emphasize preservation of anatomical structures).

Uterine incisions

Entry into the uterus can be through a midline or a transverse lower segment incision (Fig. 17.2).

Lower segment caesarean section (Fig. 17.2a)

This is the most common approach. The transverse incision is placed in the lower segment of the gravid uterus behind the utero-vesicle peritoneum.

Advantages include:

- The site is less vascular hence less blood loss.
- It contains spread of infection into abdominal cavity.
- It is in the less contractile part of the uterus hence scar rupture in subsequent pregnancy is less likely.
- Healing is better with fewer postoperative complications such as adhesions.
- Implantation of the placenta over the uterine scar is less likely in subsequent pregnancies.

Disadvantages include:

- Access may be limited.
- Proximity to the bladder increases risk of damage particularly in repeat procedures.
- Extension into the lateral angles or behind the bladder can increase blood loss.

Classical caesarean section (Fig. 17.2b)

This incision is placed vertically in the midline of the uterine body. Indications for use include:

- early gestation where the lower segment is poorly developed
- when access to the lower segment is prevented by adhesions or uterine fibroids
- when the fetus is impacted in the transverse position

- where the lower segment is vascular because of an anterior placenta praevia
- when there is cervical carcinoma
- when speed is essential, for example following death of the mother.

  Disadvantages include:

- Haemostasis is more difficult with a thick vascular incision.
- Adhesions to surrounding organs are more likely.
- The anterior placenta may be encountered during entry.
- Healing is impaired because of myometrial involution.
- There is more risk of uterine rupture in subsequent pregnancies.

Kronig–Gellhorn–Beck incision (Fig. 17.2c)

This is a midline incision in the lower segment. It is used in preterm deliveries where the lower segment is poorly formed or in situations where extension into the upper uterine segment is anticipated to provide more access. It has fewer of the complications associated with a classical caesarean section. This incision need not preclude vaginal delivery.

Other situations

An inverted T incision or a J incision may on occasion be required when access is found to be inadequate despite a lower segment incision.

These incisions are best avoided. As with classical caesarean sections, subsequent pregnancies will need to be delivered by elective caesarean section.

OPERATIVE STEPS FOR CAESAREAN SECTION

- Open the abdomen through a midline or a transverse Pfannenstiel incision. In the Pfannenstiel approach a transverse skin incision is placed above the symphysis pubis. This is followed by division of the rectus sheath and separation of the rectus muscles prior to opening the abdominal peritoneum.

- After opening the abdomen a Doyen retractor is inserted to hold the incision open for access into the lower uterine segment. Check the rotation of the uterus.
- Identify and pick up loose peritoneum (Fig. 17.3a) over the lower uterine segment and open transversely (Fig. 17.3b). Replace the Doyen retractor to displace the peritoneum and bladder away from the intended uterine incision. Avoid excessive dissection behind the bladder otherwise troublesome venous bleeding may occur.
- Incise the lower uterine segment transversely over an area of 2–3 cm until the amniotic cavity or membranes are identified. Extend the incision laterally with fingers until there is adequate room for delivery (Fig. 17.3c). Bleeding is common when the lower segment is incised and care is needed to avoid fetal damage.
- Remove the retractor. Insert a hand into the uterine wound below the breech or the fetal head (Fig. 17.3d). The presenting part is gently brought out through the uterine and abdominal incision. A characteristic hiss may be heard when the vacuum effect is lost. Facilitate delivery by fundal pressure (use the free hand or that of an assistant). An impacted presenting part can be dislodged by an assistant gently pushing through the vagina.
- Once the fetal head is delivered, clear the airways (mouth first). Carefully deliver the shoulders to avoid further extension of the incision at the lateral angles. Syntocinon (5 units) or ergotamine (0.25 mg) is given. Clamp and cut the cord. Take arterial and venous cord blood samples to assess fetal pH and base excess (particularly relevant for emergency caesarean sections). The placenta is removed manually. Ensure the uterine cavity is empty. Pass a digit through the cervical os to facilitate discharge of lochia.
- Identify lateral angles and secure bleeding vessels with clamps.
- Identify the lower edge of the uterine incision, secure the lateral angles, close the uterine wound in two layers with continuous sutures (Fig. 17.3e).

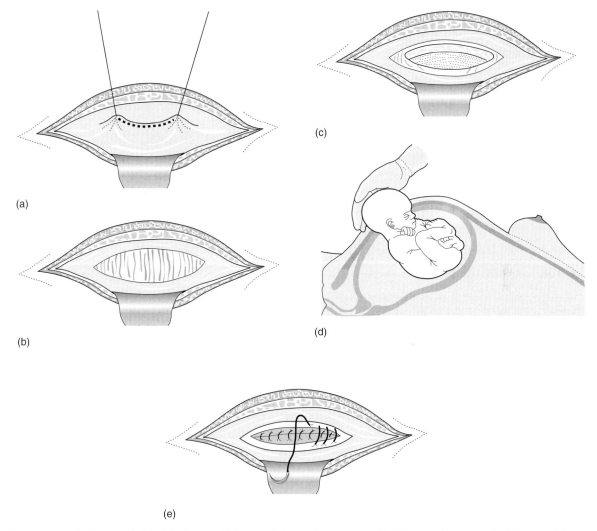

(a)

(b)

(c)

(d)

(e)

Figure 17.3 Peritoneum is (a) picked up and (b) opened, before lower segment is (c) incised transversely; fetal head (d) is delivered and uterine wound is closed (e) in two layers.

- Exteriorize the uterus if needed to facilitate uterine wound closure (warn the anaesthetist if a spinal or epidural is used for anaesthesia). When haemostasis is achieved close the peritoneum with continuous suture.
- Remove blood and clots from the peritoneal cavity. Check normality of salpinges and ovaries. Abdominal packs, if used, are removed. Use a drain if oozing is cause for concern.
- Close the abdominal wound in layers. Current practice does not require closure of the parietal peritoneum. Likewise when there is no bleeding the subcutaneous layer need not be sutured. Catgut is no longer used in contemporary surgery.
- All steps of the procedure should be clearly documented. All complications must be highlighted to support counselling for subsequent pregnancies.

See Box 17.1 for a summary of the dos and don'ts of caesarean section.

Box 17.1 Dos and don'ts of caesarean section

Do
- Place the mother in a 15° left lateral tilt (using a wedge) to overcome caval compression.
- Check the fetal heart before surgery. Operation may be contraindicated if the fetus is dead.
- If possible place the fetus into a longitudinal lie by external version.
- Once the fetus is delivered quickly the safety of the mother and her subsequent obstetric career must govern the tempo of surgery.
- The average blood loss is 400–600 ml. Consider replacement of blood if there is excessive bleeding.
- Ensure lochia can drain especially after elective caesarean section. Pass a finger or artery forceps from above through the cervix before closing the uterine incision.
- Insert drains if haemostasis is considered unsatisfactory or oozing is anticipated.
- If uterine infection is suspected take uterine swabs for culture.
- Ensure there is adequate width of the abdominal wound in a repeat transverse incision. Scar tissue is less compliant compared to normal tissue and may not stretch to allow easy delivery of the fetus.
- Thorough toilet of the abdominal cavity reduces the risk of postoperative ileus.
- Make sure uterus is contracted.
- Clean the vagina. This procedure removes a nidus for infection and allows early recognition of postoperative bleeding.
- Document clearly difficulties encountered or complications with the surgery. A plan for management of subsequent deliveries should be included.

Do not
- Do not conduct trial of labour.
- Vaginal delivery is usually contraindicated after two caesarean sections.
- Do not hesitate to use a subumbilical midline incision if a previous transverse lower abdominal incision is considered unsatisfactory.
- Avoid placing the uterine lower segment incision too close to the bladder.

CAESAREAN SECTION – SPECIFIC ISSUES

Communication

Apart from issues of consent and good practice of forewarning team members such as anaesthetists and neonatologists, it is important to define the degree of urgency for need to deliver the baby. In an emergency the current accepted decision to delivery interval is 30 minutes or less. This is, however, not an evidence based standard.

Vaginal delivery after caesarean section

Vaginal delivery is contraindicated after a classical caesarean section and if there is need to extend the transverse uterine incision (T or J incisions). Where there is no recurrent indication for caesarean section, vaginal delivery reduces maternal mortality and morbidity. There is, however, a 0.3% uterine rupture rate associated with trial of scar. There is 25% perinatal mortality and a 25% need for hysterectomy following uterine rupture (Caughey et al 1999). Although a quarter to a third of mothers with prior caesarean section can successfully deliver vaginally, the following must be satisfied:

- The mother is well and there is no obstetric complication.
- The pelvis is adequate. A trial of labour is not acceptable.
- There is no complication associated with the previous caesarean section, e.g. extension of uterine scar or infection following surgery.
- Delivery must be conducted in a safe environment where appropriate care and continuous surveillance such as fetal heart rate monitoring is available.
- A successful vaginal delivery following caesarean section need not indicate reduction in risk for a second vaginal delivery.
- The second stage should not be prolonged.

Signs of uterine scar rupture

Mothers with a classical uterine scar may experience uterine rupture prior to onset of labour. The low vertical uterine incision need not contribute increased risk to uterine rupture compared to the low transverse uterine incision. Signs of uterine rupture are:

- Fetal heart rate signs of compromise.
- Suprapubic pain present between contractions and often felt despite presence of epidural analgesia.
- There is exquisite tenderness on palpation of the lower uterine segment.
- The presence of a rising maternal pulse rate.

- There is intrapartum vaginal bleeding.
- Sudden cessation of uterine contractions.
- Abdominal palpation detects malpresentation and fetal parts are easily palpable.
- Vaginal examination may reveal the presenting part has moved up into the pelvis.
- There may be maternal shock and collapse.

Management for uterine rupture

Maternal mortality for uterine rupture was 2.3 per million maternities (DoH 1998). Correct planning of delivery and induction (judicious prostaglandin usage after one dose), delivery in an appropriate setting, and involvement of experienced obstetric staff in intrapartum care can contribute to improved outcome.

When scar rupture is suspected:

- Perform immediate laparotomy.
- After assisted delivery or during manual removal of the placenta the lower segment can be examined by an experienced surgeon. The lower segment is identified by locating the thick upper uterine segment and then withdrawing the examining finger towards the cervix. Integrity of the loose thinner lower segment is best examined by running the finger gently from side to side (Fig. 17.4). For small dehiscence with no bleeding no further action is necessary apart from close observation. Future deliveries must be by elective caesarean section. For large rupture, especially when bleeding continues, laparotomy and repair are necessary.

Caesarean section after intrauterine fetal death

This is necessary when vaginal delivery is not feasible (e.g. impacted shoulders, fetal abnormality) or for the mother's welfare (e.g. abruptio placenta, with severe bleeding and fetal death). Exclude coagulation defects. Additional psychological support will be required.

Difficulty with delivery of the fetal head

Caesarean section following a trial of labour or trial of forceps may find the fetal head impacted or deep in the pelvis. Delivery of the presenting part is facilitated by:

- Displacement of the presenting part up into the pelvis by an assistant pushing through the vagina.
- Turning the fetal head into the occipitoposterior position can assist delivery.
- Wrigley's forceps can be used. A single blade employed as a lever (Fig. 17.5) or both blades can be applied to effect delivery (Fig. 17.6). Forceps are useful to bring a high head through the uterine incision.
- Extend uterine incision e.g. inverted T (Fig. 17.7).

Caesarean hysterectomy

Indications include gross uterine rupture or uncontrollable haemorrhage. The mother is usually

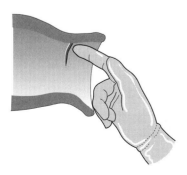

Figure 17.4 Schematic illustration of examination for uterine scar integrity.

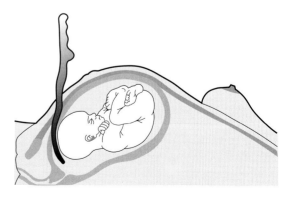

Figure 17.5 Use of single forceps blade to assist delivery of the fetal head.

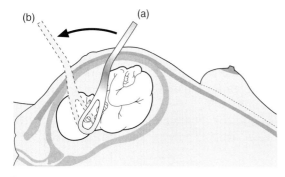

Changing the position and lifting head through uterine wall

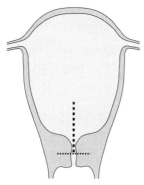

Figure 17.6 Forceps delivery in caesarean section: forceps such as Wrigley's are applied to the fetal head in the direct occipitoposterior position (a), changing to position (b), to lift head through the uterine wound and complete delivery by directing forceps towards the mother's head (c).

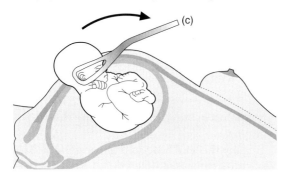

Figure 17.7 Inverted T incision.

compromised hence speed and experience are required. Consider the following:

- Time is saved if the uterus is removed before tying the pedicles after clamping.

- There may be difficulty in differentiating between the oedematous lower segment, the cervix and surrounding tissues. A subtotal hysterectomy is advised when damage and bleeding are confined to the uterine body.
- Bilateral ligation of the internal iliac artery may be required.
- Repair the ruptured uterus if the mother is stable, surgical expertise is available and fertility has to be preserved.

Classical caesarean section

Remember to check the rotation of the uterus. If possible start at the lower half of the upper uterine segment and extend if required. The uterine wall should be closed in three layers. The herringbone suture technique for closure of the superficial layer minimizes oozing.

Holding stitch

A holding stitch can help lift the lower segment away from tight application to the fetus. Traction

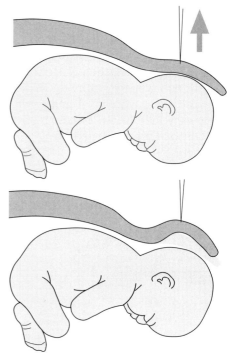

Figure 17.8 Holding stitch.

on the stitch will allow incision without damage to the fetus (Fig. 17.8). The stitch can also help identify the distal lower segment flap if difficulty is anticipated.

Bleeding lower segment uterine angles

A drier field and better control of bleeding is achieved if the uterus is delivered through the abdominal wound.

Sterilization

Consent for this procedure from both partners should be obtained well in advance. Use of an epidural or spinal anaesthesia will allow opportunities for discussion at time of surgery.

The couple should be fully counselled in terms of irreversibility of the procedure, failure rates and technique used.

The isthmic portion of salpinges are usually excised and the cut ends ligated. The excised segments should be dispensed for histological verification. Clips are less reliable when the salpinges are enlarged by pregnancy.

REFERENCES

Caughev A B, Shipp T D, Repke J T et al 1999 Rate of uterine rupture during a trial of labour in women with one or two prior Caesarean deliveries. American Journal of Obstetrics and Gynecology 181: 872–876

Department of Health 1998 Report on confidential enquiries into maternal deaths in the United Kingdom 1994–1996. HMSO, London

FURTHER READING

Appleton B, Targett C, Rasmussen M et al 2000 Vaginal birth after Caesarean section. An Australian multicentre study. VBAC study group. Australian and New Zealand Journal of Obstetrics and Gynaecology 40: 87–91

Caughev A B, Shipp T D, Repke J T et al 1999 Rate of uterine rupture during a trial of labour in women with one or two prior Caesarean deliveries. American Journal of Obstetrics and Gynecology 181: 872–876

Chazotte C, Cohen W R 1990 Catastrophic complications of previous Caesarean section. American Journal of Obstetrics and Gynecology 163: 738–742

Department of Health 1998 Report on confidential enquiries into maternal deaths in the United Kingdom 1994–1996. HMSO, London

Donald I 1979 Practical obstetric problems. Lloyd-Luke (Medical Books), London

Duff P 1987 Prophylactic antibiotics for Caesarean delivery. A simple cost-effective strategy for the prevention of post-operative morbidity. American Journal of Obstetrics and Gynecology 157: 794–798

Gregory K D, Korst L M, Cane P et al 1999 Vaginal birth after Caesarean and uterine rupture rates in California. Obstetrics and Gynecology 94: 985–989

Malkasian G D 1990 The conscience of the specialty. Obstetrics and Gynecology 75: 1–4

Martens M G, Faro S, Philips L E et al 1987 Postpartum endometritis in high risk C section patients. Infec Surg 96–99

Miller D A, Fidelia G D, Paul R H 1996 Vaginal birth after Caesarean section. New England Journal of Medicine 335: 689–695

Molmgren G, Sjoholm L, Stark M 1999 The Misgav Ladach method for caesarean section: method description. Acta Obstetrica et Gynecologica Scandinavia 78: 615–621

Per Bergsjso 1993 Quality assurance: a concept rediscovered. Acta Obstetrica et Gynecologica Scandinavia 72: 143

Shipp T D, Zelop C M, Repke J T et al 1999 Intrapartum rupture and dehiscence in patients with prior lower uterine segment vertical and transverse incisions. Obstetrics and Gynecology 94: 735–740

Sood A K et al 2000 Pregnant women with cervical cancer should be delivered by Caesarean section. Obstetrics and Gynecology 95: 832–838

Sood A K, Sorosky J I, Mayr N et al 2000 Cervical cancer diagnosed shortly after pregnancy: prognostic variables and delivery routes. Obstetrics and Gynecology 95: 832–838

18

Emergencies in the immediate puerperium

D. Liu, C. Rodeck

The exertions of labour and delivery subject mothers to potential risks (summarized in Table 18.1) because:

- Strong contractions threaten uterine rupture in any scarred uterus. Pelvic vein thrombi may be dislodged to cause pulmonary embolus and increased intrauterine pressure can squeeze amniotic fluid into the venous sinuses to produce amniotic fluid emboli. Following delivery uterine retraction injects up to 500 ml of sequestrated blood into the circulatory system. Mothers with restricted cardiac output may develop pulmonary oedema.
- Increased intra-abdominal, intrathoracic and intracranial pressures are associated with pushing efforts during delivery. Aneurysms (e.g. splenic or intracranial) or lung bullae (following chronic lung disease) can rupture.
- Placental and membrane separation expose a large area with open venous sinuses. Some bleeding is inevitable but postpartum haemorrhage can result if the myometrium fails to contract or is prevented from doing so. Occasionally a vacuum is created after expulsion of the placenta and air can be sucked in to produce air emboli.
- Mothers may react adversely to the administration of drugs such as opiates or oxytocics.
- Stress and exertion can aggravate existing medical conditions, such as epilepsy or adrenal insufficiency. A difficult labour can leave psychological sequelae.

Table 18.1 Complications resulting from strong uterine contractions

Condition	Predisposition	Signs and symptoms	Management	Prophylaxis
Uterine rupture	Uterine scarring	Range from asymptomatic to haemorrhage collapse and haemorrhage	Resuscitate, explore extent of damage and repair if indicated or perform hysterectomy	Anticipate care with oxytocics, reduce pushing in second stage, consider elective caesarean section
Pulmonary thrombo-embolism (see Box 18.1)	History of prolonged bed rest. Pelvic infection or trauma	Range from asymptomatic to pleuritic pain, blood stained sputum, dyspnoea, cyanosis and collapse	Resuscitate, ventilate, confirm diagnosis and treat with anticoagulation. ECG, blood gases and ventilation perfusion scans are helpful	Heighten index of suspicion in at-risk mothers. Aim for spontaneous delivery and short second stage. Give heparin for at-risk mothers
Amniotic fluid embolism	Polyhydramnios, excessive pushing, early placental separation, abuse of oxytocics	Collapse, dyspnoea, cyanosis, coagulation defect	Resuscitate, ventilate, hydrocortisone to treat coagulation disorder. Antibiotics	Avoid long labour and excessive pushing in mothers with predisposition. Care needed with induction of labour
Air embolism	Uterus fails to contract following rapid delivery of placenta	Sudden collapse, dyspnoea, cyanosis, cardiac arrest and 'machinery murmur'	Resuscitate, ventilate, occasionally air in right cardiac auricle or ventricle may be aspirated	Control delivery of placenta. Ensure uterine contraction
Pulmonary oedema	Restriction in cardiac output	Acute heart failure	Oxygen, digitalis, diuretics, occasionally venesection	Avoid ergometrine in at-risk mothers. Care needed if there is output obstruction

---

Box 18.1 Pulmonary thrombo-embolism

This complication remains a major cause of maternal mortality, hence prevention and correct management are important:

- Identify at-risk mothers.
- Prevention is by subcutaneous heparin 5000–10000 pre-operation and then twice daily (maintain anti-factor Xa levels below 0.3 iu/ml) or equivalent such as fragmin 2500 iu subcutaneously 1–2 hours before surgery and then daily till fully mobile to cover labour or caesarean section. Bleeding is more likely if prothrombin time is more than 2.5 times control or the heparin level exceeds 0.5 iu/ml. Pre-eclampsia, renal impairment and aspirin ingestion reduce heparin requirements.
- Mothers with anti-thrombin III deficiency are at particular risk. During labour and the early puerperium give anti-thrombin III infusions or equivalent. Heparin is not useful because its action depends on anti-thrombin III.
- Mothers with mitral valve disease or prosthetic heart valves are usually given intravenous heparin before delivery at levels of 0.8 iu/ml. Reduce levels to one-third during labour and raise again in the puerperium.
- Pulmonary embolism is often symptomless. If possible confirm diagnosis. Treatment is by heparin 40000 units daily by intravenous infusion (anti-factor Xa levels of 0.5–1.5 iu/ml; partial thrombin time PTT of 1.5–2.5 times control) for 1 week before changing regimen.
- Contraindication or caution with heparin usage includes uncontrolled hypertension, haemorrhagic disorders, peptic ulcers and advanced renal or hepatic diseases.

POSTPARTUM HAEMORRHAGE

Bleeding in excess of 300 ml after delivery is considered excessive. By convention, a loss of 500 ml or more is described as a haemorrhage.

True postpartum haemorrhage is bleeding after delivery of the placenta, an academic point of little practical value. Bleeding is further classified as primary (within 24 hours of birth) and secondary (after 24 hours after birth).

Results

- Hypovolaemic shock and death (still a major cause of maternal mortality).
- Pituitary infarct and necrosis (Sheehan's syndrome).
- Anaemia.
- Anxiety. Haemorrhage is a frightening experience and all mothers and their partners appreciate a full explanation and reassurance.

Diagnosis

- The presence of continuous fresh blood loss, torrential bleeding or collapse.
- Blood may collect in an atonic uterus with little evidence of excess external loss but fundal height increases.

Predisposing factors

- Poor maternal health.
- History of antepartum or postpartum haemorrhage.
- Prolonged labour especially after the use of oxytocics.
- Poor uterine contraction/retraction, for example in a grand multipara, or where the uterus is previously overdistended (e.g. a multiple pregnancy).
- Blood dyscrasias or inherited bleeding tendencies, for example von Willebrand's disease.
- Birth trauma, surgery and uterine inversion.
- Retained placenta or partial separation of a placenta accreta.
- An episiotomy can contribute up to 150 ml of blood loss. Episiotomies must be repaired quickly to reduce blood loss.
- Placenta praevia.

Management

- Anticipate. Set up intravenous infusion and reserve cross-matched blood for at-risk mothers. Ergometrine 0.25 mg intravenously encourages uterine contraction. Following antepartum haemorrhage coagulation defects must be excluded before delivery or surgery.
- An experienced person should conduct the delivery of at-risk mothers.
- Treat shock. Untreated severe shock for more than 30 minutes will result in Sheehan's syndrome in 40% of mothers.
- Calculate blood loss and ensure adequate replacement. Note consistency and ability of blood to clot. If necessary correct coagulation defects.

The dictum 'an empty and contracted uterus does not bleed' is worth remembering. Check size and consistency of the uterus. Removal of a blood clot in the uterine cavity may be all that is necessary.

- If the uterus is poorly contracted massage gently to encourage contraction. Place four fingers of one hand behind the fundus of the uterus with the thumb in front and massage with a circular motion (Fig. 18.1). Give 0.25 mg ergometrine intravenously if there are no contraindications such as hypertension. Maintain contraction by intravenous oxytocics (syntocinon) for 6–8 hours. A useful regimen is 20 units of syntocinon in 500 ml of physiological saline administered at 20 drops or more per minute.
- An alternative drug that produces powerful and prolonged uterine contraction is misoprostol. Rectal administration 1000 micrograms is usually highly effective.
- Intramyometrial injection of prostaglandin $F_2\alpha$ ($PGF_2\alpha$) (250 micrograms repeated in 10 minutes) can also be tried.

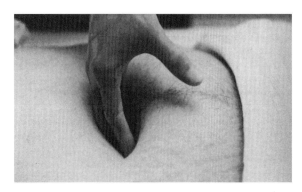

Figure 18.1 Uterine massage to encourage contraction.

- If the uterus is well contracted, conduct an exploration under adequate epidural or, preferably, general anaesthesia. Exclude vaginal, cervical or uterine lacerations. Ensure that the uterus is empty. Mothers must be observed closely for 4–6 hours after an exploratory procedure.
- Classical manoeuvres, described below, can be tried.

Bimanual compression

- Ensure adequate anaesthesia.
- Place a fist vaginally in the anterior fornix whilst the abdominal hand compresses the uterus against the fist (Fig. 18.2). This is still worth considering as a temporizing measure in torrential bleeding. It is physically exhausting and cannot be maintained for any length of time.
- Continued severe bleeding despite the above measures necessitates a hysterectomy. In a sick mother a subtotal hysterectomy is justified. Consider direct compression of the aorta (temporary measure) and ligation of the internal iliac arteries or uterine arteries where appropriate.

For mothers who may refuse blood transfusions Box 18.2 shows how this situation should be managed.

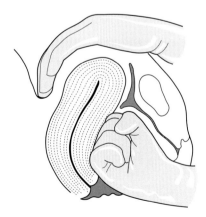

Figure 18.2 Bimanual compression of uterus.

> **Box 18.2** Management for mothers refusing a blood transfusion
>
> - Give oxygen, infuse colloid e.g. haemacel.
> - Exclude retained products of conception or trauma
> - Give syntometrine. If hypertensive give 10 u IV of syntocinon
> - Misoprostol (PGE₁ analogue) 600 micrograms oral; 800 micrograms intrauterine or 1000 micrograms rectal
> - Uterine packing
> - Brace suture
> - Hysterectomy
>
> **Postpartum**
> - IV iron sucrose (venofer) if anaemic
> - Erythropoietin 300 u/kg 3 times weekly subcutaneously helps erythropoiesis

RETAINED PLACENTA

The placenta is retained if it is not delivered within 30 minutes after the birth of the fetus. The placenta may be:

- separated but trapped by the cervix
- partially separated
- pathologically adherent (placenta accreta, increta, percreta).

Diagnosis

- A high fundus.
- Postpartum haemorrhage.
- Absent signs of placenta separation.

Management

The placenta should be removed manually (Box 18.3) if it is retained. Immediate removal is mandatory if there is haemorrhage. A hysterectomy may be required for a pathologically adherent placenta when bleeding continues.

Pathologically adherent placenta

- Incidence around 1 in 7000 pregnancies.
- MRI or transabdominal colour Doppler sonography can detect some placenta accreta and assist preoperative planning.

Box 18.3   Manual removal of placenta

- Cross-match blood. Put up drip.
- Use epidural or general anaesthesia.
- Use the lithotomy position and aseptic technique. Catheterize bladder.
- Perform a vaginal examination with liberal use of obstetric cream.
- A placenta protruding through the cervix is readily removed.
- Manual dilatation is necessary if the cervix is clamped down.
  - — Appose the tips of all five fingers of examining hand to form a cone (Fig. 18.3).
  - — Insert the tips of the fingers through cervix (Fig. 18.4).
  - — Spread the fingers repeatedly rotating hand at same time and ease the hand through the cervix (Figs 18.5 and 18.6). Stabilize the fundus with the external hand.

- Once inside the uterine cavity, locate the placenta by following the umbilical cord to its insertion.
- The placenta is separated by sliding the open hand between the placenta and the uterine wall. The abdominal hand stabilizes the uterus and acts as a guide to prevent damage to the thin myometrium (Fig. 18.7).
- Remove the placenta only when it is totally separated.
- Examine the placenta for missing cotyledons. Re-explore the uterine cavity.
- Close observation for 4–6 hours after manual removal is necessary. Make sure that the uterus is well contracted. Leave indwelling catheter.

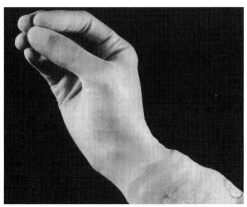

(a)

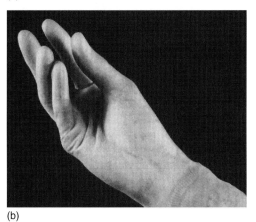

(b)

Figure 18.3   (a) Apposed fingers (b) spread repeatedly to dilate cervix.

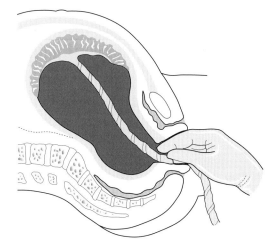

Figure 18.4   Manual dilatation of the cervix.

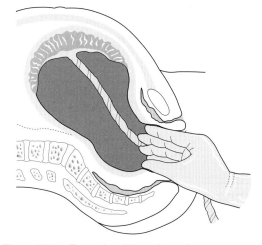

Figure 18.5   Easing hand through cervix.

Box 18.3 Manual removal of placenta *(Continued)*

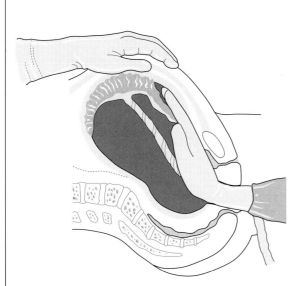

Figure 18.6 Manual removal of placenta.

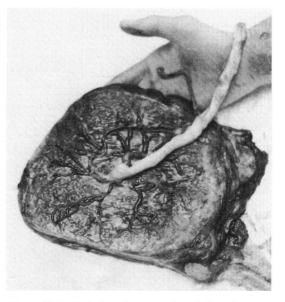

Figure 18.7 Technique for separation of placenta.

- If the placenta cannot be separated from the uterine wall, hysterectomy is often the safest option when bleeding continues. If there is no bleeding maintain close watch

and await spontaneous expulsion after some days. A pathologically adherent placenta can be left to reabsorb spontaneously. Consider use of methotrexate.

- When there is no bleeding, conservative management with use of methotrexate and close observation is an option.

ACUTE UTERINE INVERSION

The whole spectrum ranging from a dimple in the uterine fundus to complete protrusion through the introitus can present (Fig. 18.8).

Precipitating factors

- Incorrect use of fundal pressure.
- Cord traction when the uterus is not well contracted and the placenta not separated.
- Fundal insertion of the placenta.
- Uterine laxity.
- Pathological attachment of the placenta.
- Severe bearing-down efforts.
- A short cord.

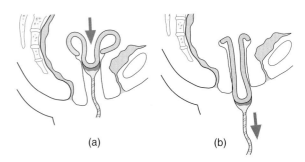

(a)   (b)

Figure 18.8 (a) Partial and (b) complete uterine inversion.

Outcome

- Shock.
- Severe dragging pain.
- Haemorrhage.
- The normal shape and position of the fundus is lost. The fundus may not be palpable but vaginal examination will confirm suspicion.

Management

- Anticipate the possibility in at-risk mothers (grand multipara, polyhydramnios).
- Prevent by proper management of the third stage of labour.
- When inversion occurs during delivery of the placenta, if the placenta is still attached replace placenta and uterus immediately. Firm pressure is applied to push the whole mass first into the vagina then through the cervix and finally into its normal position. Do not remove the placenta unless it is congested and obstructs replacement. Attempting to remove the placenta at this stage wastes time, may cause severe bleeding or may not be possible because of pathological adherence.
- Treat shock and replace blood.
- If immediate replacement is not possible general anaesthesia is necessary once the mother's condition is stabilized. Reduce the inversion gradually by applying pressure to the dependent part of the uterus, and simultaneously pressing with the other hand on all the parts of the uterus which inverted last (Fig. 18.9a, b).
- O'Sullivan's technique. The dependent part of the uterus is replaced into the vagina. Five or more litres of physiological saline are deposited into the posterior fornix of the vagina. An assistant holds the vulva against the operator's

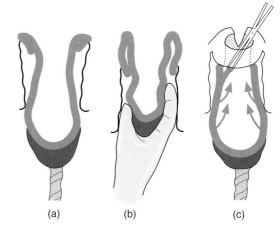

(a)   (b)   (c)

Figure 18.9   (a) and (b) Replacement of inverted uterus manually and (c) at laparotomy.

wrist or forearm to effect a watertight seal. Hydrostatic pressure replaces the uterus.
- Once the uterus is reduced, attempt to remove the placenta. Administer oxytocics to encourage contraction.
- If all attempts fail laparotomy is necessary. Incise the posterior ring of the inverted uterus to overcome resistance to replacement. Restoration to the normal position can be achieved by traction on the parts of the uterus just inside the inverted ring (Fig. 18.9c). Vaginal effort by an assistant pushing from below will help.

FURTHER READING

Chou M M, Ho E S, Lee Y H 2000 Prenatal diagnosis of placenta accreta by transabdominal colour Doppler ultrasound. Ultrasound Obstetrics and Gynecology 15: 28–35

Lemercier E, Genebois A, Descargue G et al 1999 MRI evaluation of placenta accreta treated by embolisation.

Apropos of a case. Review of the literature. Journal of Radiology 80: 383–387

O'Brien P, El-Refaey H, Gordon A et al 1998 Rectally administered misoprostol for the treatment of post partum haemorrhage unresponsive to oxytocin and ergometrine: a descriptive study. Obstetrics and Gynecology 91: 212–214

19

Malpresentation and malpositions

D. Liu

DEFINITIONS

Malposition

This describes a vertex presentation which is not in the fully flexed anterior position, for example a deflexed head, occipitolateral and occipitoposterior positions. The occiput is the denominator. A higher incidence is seen in mothers of African and Chinese origin.

Malpresentation

This describes all presentations which are not vertex, for example face, brow, shoulder and breech presentation.

ASSOCIATIONS

- Fetus: abnormal, large, preterm, multiple.
- Uterus: abnormal, polyhydramnios, poor uterine tone, pendulous abdomen.
- Pelvis: abnormal, disproportion (contracted or capacious pelvis).

LABOUR

During pregnancy attention is drawn to these complications when the fundal height does not correspond to gestational dates, the lie is not longitudinal or the fetal head is not engaged. The fetal head may appear large because it is abnormal, or is in malposition. Before or following labour, some of these complications may resolve spontaneously.

Labour in these mothers may:

- in certain circumstances produce these complications as a secondary feature (rotation from occipital anterior);
- be complicated by early membrane rupture and risk of cord prolapse;
- be prolonged or become arrested;
- require medical intervention, assisted delivery or caesarean section.

An experienced obstetrician should be called to confirm the diagnosis and then to decide about labour and supervise the mode of delivery.

Diagnosis of malpositions signals need to anticipate operative delivery.

DEFLEXED HEAD

This describes a vertex presentation where the fetal head is not fully flexed to present the most advantageous biparietal diameter of 9.5 cm. This situation arises when:

- the fetus is small in relation to the pelvis, e.g. preterm birth;
- congenital abnormalities are present;
- the dimensions of the pelvis are marginal (this is particularly likely in occipitoposterior positions);
- fibroids or tumours interfere with normal labour.

Labour is prolonged or may be arrested. Deflexion can progress to a brow or face presentation.

Delivery

Labour may be delayed in the second stage. Delivery may require an episiotomy, manual flexion of the fetal head or the application of forceps.

OCCIPITOPOSTERIOR POSITIONS

These describe the situation where the occiput is in the posterior part of the pelvis. This position is found in 10–13% of all vertex presentations. Contributory factors include:

- a large baby
- an android or anthropoid (ellipsoid) pelvis
- pelvic brim contracture or flat sacrum
- anterior low-lying placenta
- a deflexed head
- malrotation.

Diameters for consideration

- Flexed occipitoposterior: presents the sub-occipitofrontal which is 10 cm (Fig. 19.1b–c).
- Deflexed occipitoposterior: presents the occipitofrontal which is 11.5 cm (Fig. 19.1a–c).

Types

- Right occipitoposterior (ROP) is the most common, the occiput lies opposite the right sacroiliac joint.
- Left occipitoposterior (LOP).
- Direct occipitoposterior. The occiput lies in the hollow of the sacrum (Fig. 19.2).

Diagnosis

Palpation

The fetal limbs are anterior and give a hollowed appearance to the mother's lower abdomen. The head is not engaged and the sinciput is felt

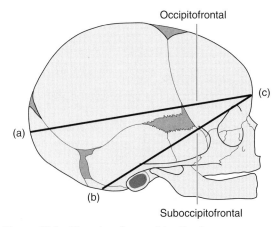

Figure 19.1 Diameters for consideration in occipitoposterior positions: occipitofrontal (a-c) and suboccipitofrontal (b-c).

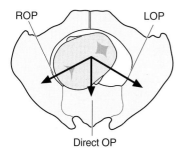

Figure 19.2 Types of occipitoposterior position: ROP, LOP and direct OP.

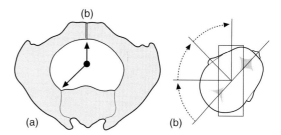

Figure 19.4 Rotation of occiput through long arc (a) to deliver in occipitoanterior position through anteroposterior diameter of outlet (b).

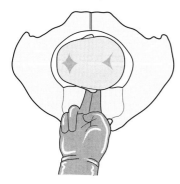

Figure 19.3 Palpating the ears as guide to direction of occiput.

superficial to the occiput when the mother, lying horizontally, is palpated. The fetal shoulder and loudest heart sounds are located well lateral to the midline.

Vaginal examination

The presenting part is poorly applied to the cervix. Deflexion is common. The anterior fontanelle is easily felt beneath the symphysis. If diagnosis presents difficulty, pass a finger alongside the fetal face and locate the ear. Running the fingers across the root of the ear will show that the pinna points in the direction of the occiput (Fig. 19.3).

Course of labour

This depends on the quality of uterine activity, whether disproportion is present and the type of pelvis.

Uterine activity

Strong regular contractions encourage flexion, engagement and rotation to an occipitoanterior position. Labour tends to be longer because the application of the presenting part of the fetus to the cervix is poor. In about two-thirds of such mothers rotation through an arc of 135° from an occipitoposterior to an occipitoanterior position will be achieved (Fig. 19.4). Extra time in labour is required to achieve this.

Gynaecoid and other adequate pelvis

Descent and flexion of the head occurs. Long rotation to the occipitoanterior position takes place at the level of the pelvic floor. Subsequent delivery is normal.

Anthropoid (ellipsoid) pelvis

Rotation to the occipitoanterior position is not favoured because the transverse diameter of the pelvis is narrow. The vertex rotates posteriorly a short distance, through 45° to deliver in the persistent occipitoposterior position. Deflexion is common, hence the presenting diameter is the wider occipitofrontal (11.5 cm) position. The head delivers by flexion followed by extension to allow the brow and the face to appear beneath the symphysis. The wider presenting diameter of the fetal head causes more trauma to the vagina, hence an episiotomy is necessary to prevent tearing. Assistance with forceps or Ventouse extraction to complete the delivery is commonly required.

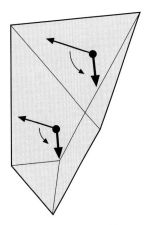

Figure 19.5 Schematic illustration of increasing difficulty for rotation to occipitoanterior in an android pelvis.

Android pelvis

Rotation to an anterior position becomes progressively more difficult with descent because the pelvis is narrow anteriorly, and the walls of the lower part of the android pelvis converge towards the outlet. Spontaneous rotation to an anterior position is possible if the pelvic diameters are adequate. In a marginal sized pelvis, failure to rotate can occur at any level of the pelvis. The vertex can remain in the occipitoposterior position or rotation may be arrested with the head in the transverse position. When failure to rotate or descend occurs deep in the pelvis, this situation is termed deep transverse arrest (DTA) (Fig. 19.5). Delivery will require assistance.

Occipitoposterior position and deflexion of the head

In a marginal sized pelvis partial deflexion will present wider fetal diameters and hence obstruction to progressive labour. With a capacious pelvis deflexion can produce a brow or face presentation.

Management

- Ensure good uterine contractions.
- Provide adequate analgesia. Epidural analgesia is useful for long labours and operative

delivery. Relaxation of the pelvic floor muscles may hinder anterior rotation.
- Assess the pelvic diameters carefully. If necessary use X-ray or perform MRI to anticipate and evaluate any likely problems.
- Avoid maternal ketosis.
- Institute close fetal surveillance.
- Examine every 2–4 hours to assess progress. Failure to progress before full cervical dilatation necessitates caesarean section. Examine immediately after membranes rupture to exclude cord prolapse.
- If the presenting part of the fetus is on the perineum in an occipitoposterior position, it is acceptable and possibly safer to deliver as an occipitoposterior with the help of an episiotomy and forceps or Ventouse extractor.
- When occipitoposterior or transverse position causes delay in the second stage the following procedures should be adopted:
  - If the presenting part of the fetus is low down assist delivery by rotation to occipitoanterior or posterior position depending on the pelvic type and ease of manoeuvre.
  - If the presenting part of the fetus is at the mid-cavity, conduct a trial of forceps rotation and delivery with preparation for caesarean section in case of failure.

FACE PRESENTATION

The incidence of face presentation is 1 in 500 deliveries. The diameter for consideration is the submentobregmatic, which is 9.5 cm. The denominator is the chin or mentum which may be found in any one of eight positions (Fig. 19.6). During labour the chin is the lowest point or leading part. Seventy-five per cent of face presentations are in the mentolateral or mentoanterior positions. Rotation in the lower half of the pelvis to the direct mentoanterior position usually occurs if the pelvis is adequate. The head is delivered by flexion. Assisted delivery is necessary for mentoposterior positions. Forceps rotation may be tried, but caesarean section is usually required for delivery (Fig. 19.7).

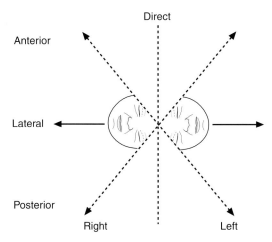

Figure 19.6   Mentum (chin) in the right and left posterior, lateral and mentoanterior positions together with direct mentoposterior and mentoanterior.

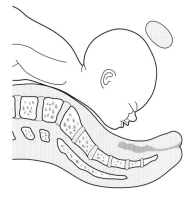

Figure 19.8   Face presentation provides situation for low presenting part with impression of non-engaged head.

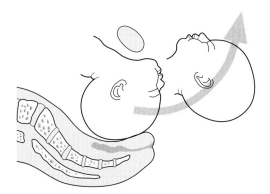

Figure 19.7   Delivery of head in mentoanterior by flexion.

Types

- Primary: face presentation before the onset of labour.
- Secondary: face presentation during the course of labour.

Diagnosis

Primary face

This is diagnosed when there is a non-engaged head, the head feels large or when the extended head is felt on the same side of the uterus as the fetal back. Radiology or ultrasound scanning is carried out to confirm suspicion. Assess adequacy of pelvis and exclude any abnormalities (fetal and maternal).

Secondary face

Suspect this diagnosis if the presenting part of the fetus appears low yet a large part of the head is palpable suprapubically. The eyes, nose, supra-orbital and alveolar ridges and the mouth can be felt on vaginal examination. Unlike the anus, the mouth does not grip the examining finger and firm fetal gums are felt. Ultrasound scan can confirm the diagnosis (Fig. 19.8).

Management

- Exclude any abnormalities. An ultrasound scan is useful.
- Assess carefully the size of the fetus and the pelvis. The face does not mould and safe vaginal delivery is not likely unless pelvic diameters are ideal.
- Ensure adequate analgesia; epidural analgesia is particularly useful.
- Maintain close surveillance. Fetal distress is likely because of the long labour and unfavourable neck positions.

Mentoanterior position

Labour is prolonged. The presenting part is poorly applied. The engaging diameter 9.5 cm

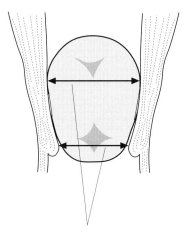

Figure 19.9 Schematic illustration to depict sequential presentation of diameter 9.5 cm twice to the cervix; first the submentobregmatic followed at right angles to this by the biparietal.

(submentobregmatic) is at a lower level than the biparietal (9.5 cm) diameter. The diameter of 9.5 cm is thus presented twice at 90° to the cervix (Fig. 19.9). With ideal conditions spontaneous delivery can occur. Usually an episiotomy and assistance with forceps are required for vaginal delivery. The Ventouse extractor is contra-indicated. Failure to progress in the first stage of labour necessitates a caesarean section.

Mentolateral position

In an adequate pelvis, expect rotation to the mentoanterior position and an assisted vaginal delivery. Rotation occurs at or below the level of the ischial spines. Manual or forceps rotation may be required. If the pelvic outlet is suspect or spontaneous rotation is arrested in mid-pelvis, deliver by caesarean section.

Mentoposterior position

Unless the fetus is very small or the pelvis capacious, the shoulder and vertex cannot be accommodated at the same time. Obstruction is inevitable. Attempting rotation to the mento-anterior position is seldom advised. Deliver by caesarean section. If the fetus is dead consider delivery by craniotomy and forceps (only if the operator is experienced). Facial oedema and bruising is usual.

BROW PRESENTATION

Brow presentation has an incidence of approximately 1 in 2000 or more deliveries.

Types

- Primary: presentation before labour. The position is usually transient and reverts to the occipitoposterior or face positions when labour starts. Exclude fetal abnormalities and inlet disproportion.
- Secondary: develops during labour. This usually follows deflexion of an occipitoposterior position.

Diameters for consideration

The fetus presents by the mentovertical diameter (13.5 cm) which is greater than the largest pelvic diameter of 12.5 cm (Fig. 19.10).

Diagnosis

Primary brow

Abdominal palpation reveals a large non-engaged head. Exclude fetal abnormality and disproportion. Await onset of labour.

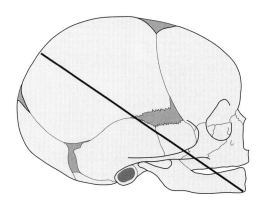

Figure 19.10 The mentovertical diameter in brow presentation.

Secondary brow

Application to the cervix is poor. The presenting part may be felt high behind the bag of fore-waters. The anterior fontanelle, supra-orbital ridge and the nose can be felt. Confirm by ultrasound scan or radiology.

Management

- If the fetus is alive and of normal size, presentation by the brow can only be safely delivered by caesarean section. Unless practised expertise is available, manipulative correction of the presentation is seldom justified.
- If the fetus is small or preterm, spontaneous delivery can occur. If assistance is necessary convert the brow to a face (mentoanterior) or occipitoposterior position before delivery by forceps.

COMPOUND PRESENTATION

This describes a situation when the hand or forearm accompanies the presenting part of the fetus. It is usually associated with poor application of the presenting part and a small or preterm infant in a large pelvis.

Management

- If compound presentation is found during labour, the hand can be pushed up behind the presenting part.
- If this is not possible, await full cervical dilatation, ensure adequate analgesia, disimpact the limb and deliver by forceps or Ventouse extraction.
- If prolapse of the whole forearm obstructs labour, a caesarean section is required.

PARIETAL PRESENTATION

In a flat pelvis the vertex engaging in the occipitolateral position will have to tilt (attitude of asynclitism) sideways to swivel past the sacral promontory and the symphysis.

Anterior asynclitism

This is when the parietal eminence in front tilts behind the symphysis. This is a favourable presentation and once the biparietal eminences swivel past the sacral promontory and symphysis, rotation to occipitoanterior or posterior is the usual course (Fig. 19.11).

Posterior asynclitism

This is when the parietal eminence at the back enters the pelvis first by slipping past the sacral promontory. This is less likely to succeed because unlike anterior asynclitism where the fetal body can lean forward anteriorly to assist engagement of the anterior parietal eminence, in posterior asynclitism the mother's spinal column prevents this action of the fetal body (Fig. 19.12). Failure of either anterior or posterior asynclitism to engage the fetal head means that a caesarean section is necessary for delivery.

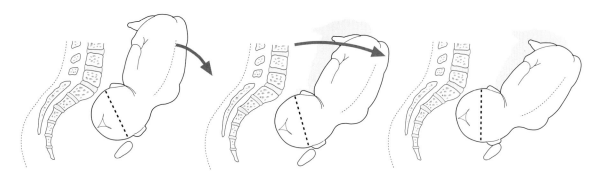

Figure 19.11   Anterior asynclitism illustrating position of fetal body to assist entry of the biparietal diameter into the pelvis.

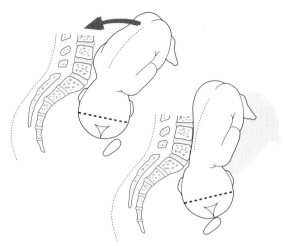

Figure 19.12 Posterior asynclitism illustrating restriction of fetal body movement to assist entry of biparietal diameter into pelvis.

SHOULDER PRESENTATION (TRANSVERSE OR OBLIQUE LIE)

In both transverse and oblique lie, the shoulder is the most common presenting part. In an oblique breech the ilium may present. Table 19.1 shows the associations of shoulder presentation.

Diagnosis

Abdomen

The fundal height appears small for dates (unless there is multiple gestation or polyhydramnios). The uterus appears broad with fullness in the flanks. No presenting part is palpable in the pelvis. The head or breech is felt opposite the iliac crest or at right angles to the midline.

Table 19.1

Maternal	Fetal
Relaxed multigravid uterus (most common cause)	Abnormality
	Twins
Pelvic contraction	Prematurity
Uterine abnormality	Fetal death
Obstruction by intra- or extrauterine masses	Polyhydramnios
	Placenta praevia

Vaginal

No vaginal examination should be performed until placenta praevia is excluded. Avoid membrane rupture and risk of cord or arm prolapse. If the membranes have ruptured, examine immediately to exclude cord prolapse. The pelvis feels empty with the ilium and/or shoulder presenting. The fetal ribs give a characteristic 'washboard' feel.

Prognosis

This is a dangerous situation for both the fetus and the mother. Spontaneous delivery is not possible unless the fetus is very small. The risk of cord prolapse, shoulder impaction, uterine rupture and the need for classical caesarean section all increase maternal and fetal mortality and morbidity.

Management

- The onset of labour with increased uterine tone may rectify the situation and convert an oblique to a longitudinal lie. This is most likely in a multigravid mother with a lax uterus.
- Identify the cause of malpresentation. Radiology or sonar examination is useful.
- Elective caesarean section is performed if vaginal delivery is contraindicated. This applies to the majority of primigravid mothers.
- If the mother is not in labour and vaginal delivery is suitable:
  — Manoeuvre fetus (external version) to longitudinal lie. This is performed in a theatre prepared for caesarean section.
  — Set up intravenous oxytocin to generate and maintain uterine contractions.
  — Perform amniotomy, drain liquor slowly and guide the presenting part into the pelvis.
- If the mother is in early labour with ruptured membranes:
  — Perform vaginal examination to exclude prolapse of the limbs or cord.
  — Attempt to encourage a longitudinal lie if vaginal delivery is considered possible. If

this is not successful deliver by caesarean section. A midline abdominal incision followed by a low vertical incision in the uterus is advised when fetal lie is fixed. Convert the vertical uterine incision to a classical incision if necessary.

- Impacted shoulders. Whether the fetus is alive or dead, deliver by caesarean section. Destructive procedures in inexperienced hands may result in uterine rupture.
- Spontaneous expulsion of the fetus can only occur if the fetus is macerated or is very small.

FURTHER READING

Gardber G M, Laakkonen E, Salevarra M 1998 Sonography and persistent occiput posterior position: a study of 408 deliveries. Obstetrics and Gynecology 91: 746–749

Gardber G M, Tuppurainen M 1994 Persistent occiput posterior presentation – a clinical problem. Acta Obstetrica et Gynecologica Scandinavica 73: 45–47

Holmberg N G, Lilieqvist B, Magnusson S, Segerbrand E 1977 The influence of the bony pelvis in persistent occiput posterior position. Acta Obstetrica et Gynecologica Scandinavica Suppl 66: 49–54

To W W K, Li I C F 2000 Occipital posterior and occipital transverse positions: reappraisal of obstetric risks. Australian and New Zealand Journal of Obstetrics and Gynaecology 40: 275–279

20

Breech

D. Liu, P. Loughna

The presenting part of the fetus is the breech with the sacrum as the denominator. It is more common before 28 weeks (20% incidence) than at term (3%). Associated causes such as disproportion, obstructing pelvic masses (e.g. fibroids, ovarian cysts), uterine abnormalities (e.g. septate uterus), hydramnios, fetal prematurity or abnormalities and multiple gestation will influence the management of labour. Breech presentation is a marker for potential fetal handicap since it is more common in preterm and structurally abnormal fetuses.

DIAGNOSIS

- The fetal head is palpated above the umbilicus.
- Fetal heart sounds are heard most easily above the umbilicus, or if heard suprapubically, the heart sound becomes louder as one progresses towards the uterine fundus.
- Fetal movements are felt maximally away from the fundus.
- Diagnosis is confirmed by ultrasonography or vaginal examination (provided placenta praevia is excluded).

Vaginal examination

- Palpate the soft buttocks and three firm areas: the fetal sacrum and two ischial tuberosities.
- In labour, once the membranes are ruptured, the baby's feet may be felt. Differentiate from the hand by feeling five even-length digits at the end of the limb and by recognizing the heel.

- Unlike the mouth, the fetal anus, when gently depressed, will grip the examining finger. Meconium may be present when the finger is withdrawn.

CLASSIFICATION

The presentation is governed by the position of the lower limbs. Sometimes the lie may be more oblique than longitudinal.

Extended (frank) (Fig. 20.1a)

This is the most common, occurring in 75% of primigravid and 50% of multigravid breeches. Good application to the cervix is possible but the extended legs may act as splints affecting the lateral flexion of the body. Delivery of the legs requires assistance.

Flexed (complete or full) (Fig. 20.1b)

This occurs mainly in multigravid mothers with good pelvic diameters or in multiple gestation. There is a risk of cord prolapse. Spontaneous or easy delivery of lower limbs is likely.

Footling or knee (incomplete) (Fig. 20.1c)

This is uncommon. There is poor application to the cervix, hence a higher risk of cord prolapse. It may indicate difficulty in engagement, thus delivery by caesarean section is recommended.

ANTENATAL ASSESSMENT

- Confirm presentation by ultrasound. This will permit description of the type of breech presentation. Vaginal delivery is acceptable only for frank or complete breech.
- Perform ultrasound biometry to gain an estimated fetal weight. Check for fetal abnormality, liquor volume and placental site. Exclude hyperextension of the fetal head.
- If gestation is uncomplicated, 37 weeks or more and not in labour, offer external cephalic version (ECV) (Box 20.1). This involves turning the baby to a cephalic presentation by gentle manual rotation, with or without tocolysis. If the procedure is performed on a Rhesus negative mother, anti-D should be administered. ECV is most likely to be successful in a flexed

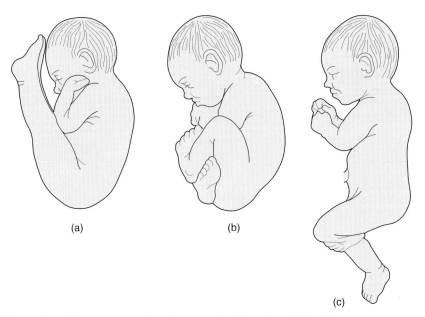

(a) (b) (c)

Figure 20.1 Breech presentation (a) extended, (b) flexed and (c) footling.

breech that is not engaged in the pelvis, when liquor is adequate and in multiparous mothers. Facilities for immediate caesarean section must be available. Epidural anaesthesia can increase success rates of ECV.

- If ECV is declined or unsuccessful, the mode of delivery needs to be discussed. Factors which should be considered include the estimated fetal weight, clinical pelvimetry, relative risks of caesarean section versus vaginal breech delivery (see below), and mother's informed options.
- ECV for preterm breech is not justified.
- In preterm breech delivery seek informed opinion of parents to determine mode of delivery. There is insufficient evidence to support use of caesarean section for all preterm deliveries.
- Where appropriate vaginal delivery of the non-vertex second twin is still acceptable.

SPONTANEOUS BREECH DELIVERY

The widest part of the pelvic brim is usually the transverse diameter whereas the anteroposterior diameter is the widest part of the pelvic outlet. In spontaneous delivery the three fetal diameters, the bitrochanteric, bisacromial and anteroposterior of the fetal head, enter in sequence through the pelvic brim in the transverse or oblique diameter and are then guided by the levator ani muscles to fit the anteroposterior diameter of the outlet.

The breech enters the pelvis with the trochanters aligned in the transverse or oblique diameter of the brim. Rotation takes place so the bitrochanteric diameter delivers through the anteroposterior diameter of the outlet. Once delivered, the breech rotates to the sacroanterior position so that the shoulders enter in the transverse diameter of the brim. Internal rotation allows the delivery of the shoulders in the anteroposterior position of the outlet and the passage of the head through the brim in the occipitolateral position. Following delivery of the shoulders (anterior shoulder delivers first), aided by lateral flexion of the trunk, the sacrum again rotates anteriorly so the posteroanterior diameter of the head (with the occiput beneath the symphysis pubis) delivers by flexion in the anteroposterior

---

Box 20.1   External cephalic version (ECV)

General points
- Vaginal term breech delivery is associated with perinatal mortality and morbidity rates between 1 and 2%. The calculated excess risk of neonatal death is about 4 per 1000. Some 70% of term breeches are delivered by caesarean section.
- Between 60 and 70% (range 50–80%) ECVs at term are successful. Up to 75% of these can deliver vaginally in cephalic presentation. ECV can reduce the overall caesarean section rate by 1%.

Contraindications
- Intrauterine growth restriction
- Multiple pregnancies
- Maternal obstetric complications
- Fetal compromise
- Oligohydramnios (amniotic fluid below 5 cm)
- Polyhydramnios (amniotic fluid over 25 cm)
- High body mass index
- Previous caesarean section
- Established labour or ruptured membranes
- Nuchal cord
- Conditions necessitating caesarean section.

Procedure for ECV
- Ensure gestation is 37 or more weeks.
- Provide detailed counselling. Obtain consent.
- Perform ultrasound scan and exclude contraindications.
- Obtain cardiotocographic trace.
- Dispense tocolytic (ritodrine 0.3 mg intravenously 2–3 minutes) if necessary.
- Check maternal heart rate is less than 120 beats per minute if ritodrine is used.
- Place mother in a 30° lateral tilt.
- Use gentle pressure to direct fetal head into pelvis. Apply pressure for 5 minutes at each attempt. Auscultate to check heart rate. Abandon procedure if mother complains of discomfort.

Post procedure
- Administer anti-D (500 iu) for Rhesus negative mothers (up to 5% small feto-maternal bleeds) if indicated by Kleihauer test.
- Repeat ultrasound scan and trace fetal heart rate for 30 minutes (some 8% may show transient fetal heart rate changes).
- Mother can go home if there is no complication.
- Perform check scan in a week to determine fetal presentation and lie.
- If ECV failed rediscuss mode of delivery. There is a place for elective caesarean section since vaginal delivery is more hazardous.

---

diameter of the pelvis. Figure 20.2 gives the possible positions of breech presentation.

Figure 20.3a shows the delivery of the breech and rotation of the sacrum anteriorly to assist the

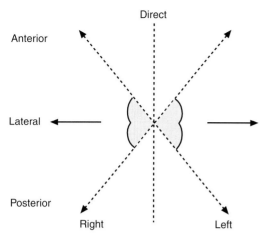

Figure 20.2 Breech presentation in the eight positions of the right and left sacroanterior, lateral and posterior together with direct sacroanterior and posterior.

entry of the shoulders through the brim while Figure 20.3b shows the restitution of the sacrum to the lateral position to allow the shoulders to deliver in the anteroposterior diameter of the pelvic outlet. Meanwhile the fetal head enters the transverse diameter of the brim. Figure 20.3c shows that after delivery of the shoulders the back rotates to the anterior position again to allow anteroposterior diameters of the fetal head to deliver through the anteroposterior diameter of the outlet.

See Box 20.2 for assisted breech delivery.

Dangers in breech delivery

- Perinatal morbidity and mortality is up to nine times higher than that for spontaneous vertex delivery. The incidence of trauma and hypoxic damage is particularly high in small preterm babies (under 1.5 kg) and in big babies (over 3.5 kg). It must be remembered that more preterm and abnormal babies present by the breech.
- The likelihood of cord prolapse (5%) and cord compression is increased.
- The head is the widest and least compressible part of the fetus. The head may be trapped if the cervix is not fully dilated (especially in preterm infants) or if there is outlet contracture of the pelvis leading to hypoxia. There is little or no time for moulding hence the pelvic diameters must be more than just adequate to ensure safe delivery.
- There is an increased likelihood of placental separation in the second stage because of traction on the cord.
- There is increased maternal risk. If an epidural or spinal anaesthetic is not in place there is increased requirement for general anaesthesia. Assistance with delivery is more likely.

There is an increasing trend for breeches to be delivered by elective caesarean section, with the result that the number of operators skilled in vaginal delivery is reduced. However, the steps

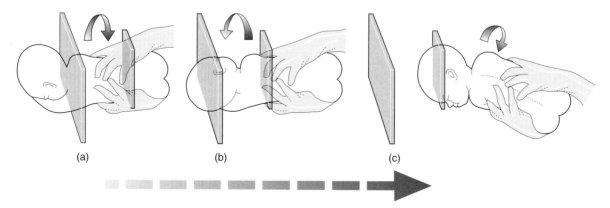

(a)   (b)   (c)

Figure 20.3 Geometric representation of breech delivery through the wide transverse/oblique diameter at the brim and the anteroposterior of the outlet. Delivery of the bitrochanteric (a), the bisacromial (b), and sagittal suture (c) are shown in sequence.

Box 20.2 Assisted breech delivery

- It is useful for the operator to have an assistant who is scrubbed.
- Most breech deliveries require minimal gentle assistance by the operator.
- The mother should be placed in the lithotomy position, with her bottom just overlapping the edge of the bed. She should be encouraged to push as for vertex presentation.
- An episiotomy is usually necessary, but should not be performed until the fetal anus is visible on the perineum.
- If there is any delay in spite of good maternal effort apply gentle groin traction. The operator's fingers must be directed into the groin to avoid fracturing the thigh or dislocating the hips (Fig. 20.4a).
- Allow the trunk to deliver in the sacrolateral position until the tip of the anterior scapula appears beneath the symphysis. The operator should support the breech, rather than apply traction.
- The legs will deliver spontaneously or readily with a little help. For extended legs deliver the anterior leg first (Fig. 20.4b). Abduct the thigh, flex the knee, secure the foot and guide it out of the pelvis by bringing it across the fetal trunk. Repeat this manoeuvre for the posterior leg. Free a loop of cord to avoid tension on it.
- Place a towel or dry cloth over the baby's pelvis to prevent the hand slipping. Grasp the pelvis with both hands. Place the hands low down to avoid damage to the fetal liver or spleen. The thumbs are placed over the sacrum.
- Apply Lovsett's manoeuvre to deliver the arms. Firm

downward traction is applied whilst rotating the fetal trunk through 180° to bring the posterior shoulder to lie anteriorly. When the elbow appears beneath the symphysis, that arm (and hand) is delivered by sweeping it across the fetal body. While maintaining gentle downward traction rotate 180° in the reverse direction to deliver the second shoulder. These manoeuvres may need to be repeated.

- Figure 20.5a shows Lovsett's manoeuvre to deliver the posterior shoulder, and Figures 20.5b and c show delivery of the anterior shoulder. Lovsett's manoeuvre depends on a short symphysis and a long curved sacrum. Traction and 180° rotation delivers point Y. Further traction and reverse rotation through 180° delivers point X.
- Once the shoulders are delivered maintain progress by gentle traction on the ankles with both hands, until the hairline appears. Raise legs through an arc until the body is vertical to the maternal spine. This technique (Burns–Marshall) flexes the fetal head and places it in the anteroposterior diameter of the pelvic outlet (Fig. 20.6). The baby's head may deliver spontaneously with this manoeuvre so care should be taken to anticipate delivery.
- If the head is not delivered, clear airways. Suck out the pharynx first. Forceps can be applied directly to assist the delivery of the head (after-coming head) (Fig. 20.7). Mauriceau–Smellie–Veit manoeuvre may be used as an alternative method for delivery of the fetal head (Fig. 20.8).

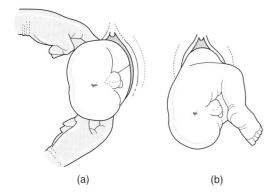

(a)   (b)

Figure 20.4 Groin traction (a) and delivery of anterior leg (b).

employed in the delivery of a breech at caesarean section are similar to those employed in vaginal delivery, hence caesarean section deliveries provide some teaching opportunities.

Labour

- Careful monitoring of fetal wellbeing and progress of labour are important. Direct fetal heart rate monitoring is feasible by the application of a fetal scalp electrode to the fetal buttock, taking care to avoid the external genitalia.
- Cord compression or cord entanglement is more common. Cord compression patterns are therefore likely. Fetal blood sampling can be performed if indicated, with the region around the ischial tuberosity being the best site for blood sampling. It is often necessary to press the blade firmer to ensure a flow of capillary blood.
- Epidural anaesthesia may facilitate maternal cooperation during the second stage.
- Induction and augmentation of labour are acceptable in selected situations.
- Suboptimal care is the most frequent cause of intrapartum fetal death and stillbirth.

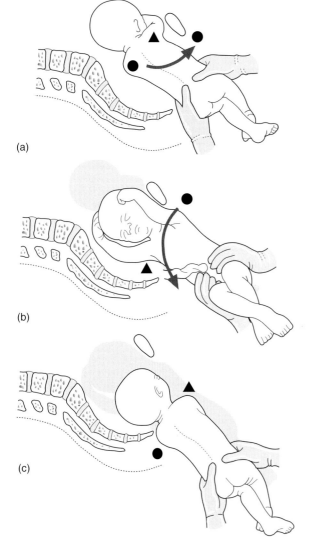

(a)

(b)

(c)

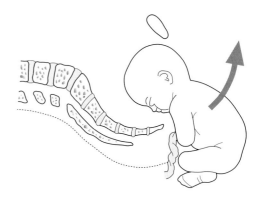

Figure 20.6 Burns–Marshall technique. Grasp legs, apply gentle traction, lift through an arc.

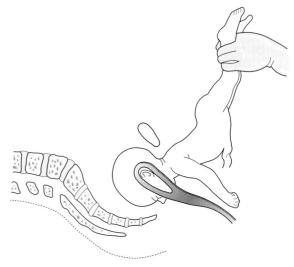

Figure 20.7 Delivery of the after-coming head by forceps.

Figure 20.5 Lovsett's manoeuvre to deliver the arms. Technique depends on the presence of a short symphysis and a long curved sacrum. Rotation through 180° and traction delivers the posterior shoulder (a). Second rotation (b) in reverse direction delivers the anterior shoulder (c). Repeat manoeuvre if necessary.

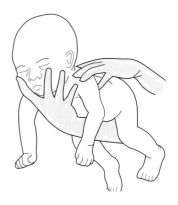

Figure 20.8 Placement of hands in the Mauriceau–Smellie–Veit technique. The infant's body is straddled on the forearm with index and middle fingers placed on malar processes to encourage flexion. Place free hand over shoulders, allowing middle finger to press on the occiput to encourage flexion. Apply downward pressure and lift body upwards when occiput appears beneath symphysis to deliver the face, brow and vertex.

- Delivery must be by an experienced member of staff. Maintain competence by breech delivery drills.

DOS AND DON'TS WITH BREECH DELIVERY

Box 20.3 summarizes the dos and don'ts of breech delivery.

BREECH IN THE SECOND TWIN OR TRIPLET

- It is acceptable to deliver the breech second twin vaginally if conditions are satisfactory.
- After delivery of the first twin the assistant places the breech or non-vertex positions into longitudinal lie (external version).
- Ensure continuing uterine contractions with a syntocinon infusion if necessary. If the breech is at the level of the ischial spine or lower, rupture the membranes between contractions and allow the liquor to drain.

- Spontaneous breech delivery is anticipated in the next few contractions.
- If the breech is high in the pelvis or still in an oblique position, rupture the membranes, locate and bring the anterior leg down (internal podalic version, Fig. 20.9).
- Delivery is accomplished by breech extraction where the obstetrician actively passes the breech through the steps required for delivery.

DELIVERY BY CAESAREAN SECTION

- Check that the breech is in longitudinal lie.
- For a footling breech first deliver the anterior then the posterior leg.
- In a flexed or extended breech, the baby's bottom is lifted out through the uterine incision with the breech in the sacrolateral position. Groin traction is then applied to deliver the trunk until the tip of the anterior scapula is visible. Extended legs are delivered as previously described.

Box 20.3   Breech delivery – dos and don'ts

Do

- Learn how to deliver a breech. To perform a caesarean section just because the second twin is a breech is bad obstetric practice.
- Follow the dictum – breech plus obstetric complication justifies caesarean section.
- Use lithotomy position. The mother's bottom should just overlap the edge of the bed. Have serum grouped and saved. Both the anaesthetist and the paediatrician should be present before delivery commences.
- If the mother wishes a vaginal delivery and clinical measurements are suspect request pelvimetry (MRI or a CT scan).
- Consider delivery of the preterm breech (<1500 g) or a fetus with an estimated fetal weight of more than 3500 g by caesarean section. The perinatal mortality doubles with vaginal breech deliveries over 3600 g and increases with increasing weight. Below 1500 g the mortality is halved if caesarean section is used.
- Vaginal breech deliveries must be managed to minimize risk of hypoxia. Once the breech is delivered to the umbilicus the rest of the fetus should be delivered in 10 minutes or less. Monitor the fetal heart rate closely during all breech deliveries.
- Perform a vaginal examination once the membranes have ruptured to exclude cord prolapse.
- Realize that, although descent of the presenting part

may be slow, in an adequate pelvis total labour time should be similar to that in cephalic presentation.
- Observe progress of the labour carefully if oxytocics are used. Augmentation of labour without due care is associated with increased perinatal mortality and morbidity.
- Consider a caesarean section for dysfunctional uterine action associated with breech presentation.

Do not
- Do not conduct trial of labour in a breech if pelvic diameters are suspect. Caesarean section is the safest mode of delivery in such situations.
- Do not attempt delivery without some experience or without supervision by an experienced obstetrician.
- Do not let the breech hang from the vulva after delivery of the shoulders. This procedure is of little value and increases the risk of hypoxic insult to the fetus.
- Delay in descent of the breech after full cervical dilatation (i.e. delay in the second stage) is an indication for caesarean section. Do not use oxytocics. Breech extraction is rarely justified, except in the delivery of a second twin which is equal or smaller in size compared with the first twin.
- Do not attempt breech extraction unless experienced.
- Do not apply traction on the jaws in the Mauriccau Smellie–Veit technique as dislocation or fracture of the mandible may result.

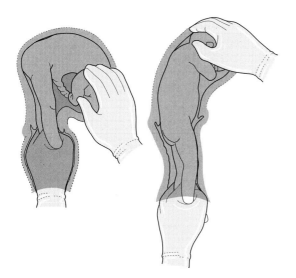

Figure 20.9   Internal podalic version.

- Lovsett's technique is used to deliver the arms.
- After delivery of the arms the obstetrician faces the mother's head and places the baby in longitudinal lie with the back uppermost. The ankles are grasped and whilst tension is maintained the trunk is directed through a 90° arc similar to the Burns–Marshall technique. Do not hyperflex the neck. Clear the airways.
- Whilst one hand holds the baby in the upright position, the baby's head can be lifted out with the free hand. If difficulty is encountered the assistant holds the breech whilst Wrigley's forceps are applied directly to the after-coming head to effect delivery.
- In preterm infants of 30 weeks or less gestation the fetal head may be considerably larger than the trunk. The lower uterine segment is poorly formed and a transverse incision in the lower segment of the uterus may not be adequate for atraumatic delivery of the preterm breech. The low vertical uterine incision (Kronig's incision) is advised. Classical caesarean section may be considered.

SPECIAL SITUATIONS

- The cervix is not fully dilated – this usually occurs in preterm deliveries. Deliver by firm downward traction with the baby's back uppermost. Digital pressure on the malar processes assists flexion. Consider using forceps. In extreme circumstances, it may be necessary to cut the cervix at 10 and 2 o'clock positions (avoiding the lateral blood vessels) using scissors. The cervix is sutured after delivery is completed.
- When there is disproportion of the fetal head, e.g. in the hydrocephalic baby, vaginal delivery can be achieved after decompression of the head. If the baby is normal and alive, symphysiotomy or caesarean section are the only avenues for a live birth.

Box 20.4   Preterm breech

- 25% incidence between 24 and 32 weeks gestation.
- Higher incidence of congenital abnormality, poor growth, lower fetoplacental ratio and perinatal complications.
- Perform ultrasound scan to confirm diagnosis, exclude congenital abnormality, assess fetal weight and check placental site.
- Determine if delivery is imminent, essential or can be delayed by tocolytics for corticosteroid administration or transfer to specialist centres.
- Discuss fully options, risks and merits of delivery modes with mothers and their partners.
- Occipital disasters with resultant cerebellar damage, intra- or periventricular damage following haemorrhage or ischaemia, or trauma to body, limbs and internal organs can occur with vaginal delivery or caesarean section.

- Deliveries should be attended by an experienced obstetrician, anaesthetist and paediatrician.
- Vaginal delivery needs particular attention to umbilical cord prolapse (especially if footling breech presentation) and incomplete cervical dilatation trapping fetal head (delivery by flexion of the head or rarely cervical incisions at 10 and 2 or 4 and 8 o'clock). Use of forceps for the after-coming head is controversial.
- Caesarean section may need a lower segment midline incision (Kronig or DeLee incision) or classical section because the lower uterine segment is poorly formed. Mothers must be made aware of increased morbidity following midline or classical section and need for repeat caesarean section to avoid threat of uterine rupture.
- Competency of neonatal support must be considered when mode of delivery is discussed.

- Face to pubes position – gently rotate the baby through 180° to bring the occiput to the anterior position and deliver as previously described. If the head is well down rotation may exert too much pressure on the fetal neck.

Apply forceps to the head after the Burns–Marshall manoeuvre.

Box 20.4 describes management of preterm breech.

FURTHER READING

Bingham P, Lilford R J 1987 Management of the selected term breech presentation: assessment of the risk of selective vaginal delivery versus Caesarean section for all cases. Obstetrics and Gynaecology 69: 965–978

Cheng M, Hannah M 1993 Breech delivery at term: a critical review of the literature. Obstetrics and Gynaecology 82: 605–618

Hannah M E, Hannah W J, Henson J A et al 2000 Planned Caesarean section versus planned vaginal birth for breech presentation at term: a randomised multicentre trial. Lancet 356: 1375–1383

Hofmeyr G J 1991 ECV at term; how high the stakes? British Journal of Obstetrics and Gynaecology 93: 1–3

Hytten F E 1982 Breech presentation: is it a bad omen? British Journal of Obstetrics and Gynaecology 89: 879–880

International Federation of Gynaecology and Obstetrics (FIGO) 1995 Recommendations of the committee on perinatal health on guidelines for the management of breech delivery. European Journal of Obstetrics and Gynaecology and Reproductive Biology 58: 89–92

Laros R K, Dattel B J 1988 Management of twin pregnancy: the vaginal route is still safe. American Journal of Obstetrics and Gynecology 158: 1330–1338

Lau T K, Lo K W K, Wan D, Rogers M S 1997 The implementation of external cephalic version at term for singleton breech presentation – how can we further increase its impact? Australian and New Zealand Journal of Obstetrics and Gynaecology 27: 393–396

Mancuso K M, Yancey M K, Murphy J A, Markenson G R 2000 Epidural analgesia for cephalic version: a randomised trial. Obstetrics and Gynaecology 95: 648–651

Rosen M G, Debanne S, Thompson K, Bilenker R M 1985 Long term neurological morbidity in breech and vertex births. American Journal of Obstetrics and Gynecology 151: 718–720

Royal College of Obstetricians and Gynaecologists 1998 Pelvimetry – clinical indications. Guideline Number 14, RCOG Press, London

Saunders N J, St G 1996 Breech delivery in the United Kingdom at the end of this century. Contemporary Review in Obstetrics and Gynaecology 8: 82–85

Society of Obstetricians and Gynaecologists of Canada 1994 Policy statement: the Canadian consensus on breech management at term. Journal of the Society of Obstetricians and Gynaecologists of Canada 16: 1839–1858

Viegas O A C, Ingemarsson I, Low P S et al 1985 Collaborative study on preterm breeches: vaginal delivery versus Caesarean section. Asia Oceania Journal of Obstetrics and Gynaecology 11: 349–355

Wallace R L, Schifrin B S, Paul R H 1984 The delivery route for very low birthweight infants. Journal of Reproductive Medicine 29: 736–740

Wigglesworth J S, Husemeyer R P 1977 Intra cranial birth trauma in vaginal breech delivery: the continued importance of injury to the occipital bone. British Journal of Obstetrics and Gynaecology 84: 684–691

21

Twins and multiple deliveries

D. Liu

Multiple pregnancy is the term used when there is more than one fetus in the uterine cavity. Twins describes two fetuses, triplets three fetuses and so on. The incidence of twinning is 40 per 1000 births for West Africans, 12 per 1000 for Caucasians and 6 per 1000 for Asians. The twinning rate is higher in fertile and older multiparous women. The advent of assisted fertility therapy increases the incidence of multiple pregnancies.

TYPES

Monozygotic or monochorionic twins (uniovular/monovular/identical)

These are produced when one ovum divides to form two fetuses (Fig. 21.1a). They can be dichorionic diamniotic, monochorionic diamniotic or monochorionic monoamniotic. The monozygotic twinning rate of 3–5 per 1000 is similar for all ethnic groups. (The fetal sex is always the same.) Complications such as hydramnios, fetal

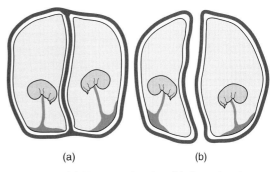

(a)   (b)

Figure 21.1   (a) Monozygotic twins, (b) dizygotic twins.

abnormality, discrepancy in fetal weight and fetal transfusion syndrome are more likely, as are intrapartum complications and poor perinatal outcome. When one twin dies in utero there is a 25% risk of necrotic neurological and renal lesions and intrauterine death in the survivor.

Dizygotic twins (binovular, non-identical)

With dizygotic twins two ova are shed, usually in the same menstrual cycle, and fertilized by two different sperms (Fig. 21.1b). The fetal sex often differs. Twinning rate differs in different ethnic groups and is influenced by the use of fertility drugs to induce ovulation.

Other multiples

These are seldom monovular; they usually follow multiple ovulation or combinations of monovular and multiple ovulation.

DIAGNOSIS

Diagnosis before delivery is important. Undiagnosed twins present additional risks to the mother and to the second fetus.

Perform ultrasound scans for all mothers with a family history of twins or where fertility drugs have been prescribed. The following factors should alert the obstetrician to the possibility of twin pregnancy:

- The uterus is large for dates or there is a history of acute hydramnios (complicates 12% of twin pregnancies).
- The mother describes fetal movement felt all over the uterus.
- Palpation of more than two fetal poles (head and breech), a small head in a large uterus or multiple fetal parts.
- Simultaneous detection of two fetal heart beats with rates differing by 10 beats or more per minute.
- Preterm labour where the uterus is larger than dates. Twins are five times more likely to be born preterm than singletons, especially before 32 weeks.

When multiple pregnancy is suspected confirm by sonar scanning. Undiagnosed twins are unlikely when there are programmes of routine antenatal ultrasound scanning. Chorionicity should be determined. This is 100% accurate in first trimester and 80–90% in mid-trimester using ultrasound for scanning.

PRESENTATION AT DELIVERY

Malpresentation and malposition especially in the second twin are common, hence the high incidence of assisted or operative deliveries. In 75% the first twin presents by the vertex, but abnormal presentation occurs in over 50% of twin deliveries.

Frequency of combinations of presentation

- Vertex/vertex – 45%
- Vertex/breech – 25%
- Breech/vertex – 10%
- Breech/breech – 9%
- Vertex/transverse – 11%
- Breech/transverse – 11%
- Transverse/transverse – 11%

COMPLICATIONS OF TWIN PREGNANCY AND DELIVERY

Pre-eclampsia (20%), uterine atony, anaemia and a large placenta increase the likelihood of post-partum haemorrhage. Cross-match and reserve blood when mothers are admitted into the labour ward. An increased rate of congenital abnormalities (twice as common and includes cardiac anomalies, bowel atresia, neural tube defects), intrauterine growth retardation (30%) and preterm labour and delivery (10% before 34 weeks, 40% before 37 weeks) contribute to the higher perinatal mortality of 3–5%. Up to three-quarters of perinatal losses are due to delivery before 34 weeks. Compared with singleton pregnancies cerebral palsy is eight times greater in twin and 47 times greater in triplet pregnancies.

First twin

First twin has a higher perinatal mortality than with singleton births because of prematurity, cord prolapse, fetal abnormality and birth injury (double the singleton rates).

Second twin

With the second twin malpositions, malpresentations, prolonged delivery interval, likelihood of placental separation and greater need for operative delivery result in lower Apgar scores. The neonatal mortality, mainly due to birth trauma, is twice that of the first twin. The danger of hypoxia increases the risk of cerebral palsy in the second twin.

In general the perinatal mortality rate of twins is 4–5 times that of singletons. Mortality due to asphyxia is 5 times that of singletons. Risk of stillbirth between 37 and 42 weeks is 6–9 per 1000 births. Delivery at 38 weeks is advised.

VAGINAL DELIVERY OR CAESAREAN SECTION

The high incidence of prematurity together with the risk of hypoxia and damage in the second twin mean that vaginal delivery is only safe when conditions are ideal. Accurate knowledge of gestational dates and the fetal weight is important. Ultrasound examination forewarns of fetal abnormalities. A lateral erect pelvimetry or better still magnetic resonance imaging of the pelvis is advised if clinical pelvic assessment suggests reduced pelvic diameters. In general vaginal delivery is preferred for vertex–vertex presentation.

Vaginal delivery may be contemplated if:

- there is no obstetric complication
- reliable monitoring of both fetal heart rates is achieved
- gestation is 32 weeks or the fetal weight is 1500 g or more.

Caesarean section is advisable if:

- there are obstetric complications or evidence of poor intrauterine growth, particularly in the second twin
- the first twin is in a breech presentation and/or gestation is less than 32 weeks
- there is abnormal presentation of the first twin

- maternal pelvic diameters are reduced
- after a previous caesarean section.

For the breech second twin, if acceptable to the informed mother vaginal breech delivery is only advised if conditions are suitable and an experienced obstetrician is present. Likewise for the non-vertex second twin, internal podalic version followed by breech extraction when conditions are suitable is the advised primary procedure. Elective caesarean section is a recognized option.

Box 21.1 describes the procedure for delivery.

Box 21.1   Delivery of twins

- Place the mother in the lithotomy position with a left lateral tilt.
- Make available forceps and Ventouse extractor especially if the second twin presents by the vertex.
- Consider an intravenous drip with syntocinon (e.g. 5 units in 500 ml of normal saline).
- An episiotomy is usually advisable.
- Maintain continuous monitoring of the second twin in the second stage.
- Deliver the first twin in the normal fashion for vertex position. If presentation is occipitoposterior, rotation to occipitoanterior may be difficult hence may necessitate delivery as a direct occipitoposterior presentation. The fetus is frequently smaller and delivery as a direct occipitoposterior presentation gives little difficulty.
- After delivery of the first twin clamp the cord, palpate the abdomen and ensure that the second twin is in the longitudinal lie. Perform external version if appropriate.
- Run syntocinon at 20–40 drops/minute to maintain uterine contractions.
- Rupture the membranes of the second sac. Perform internal podalic version if appropriate.
- The vertex or breech presentation usually delivers readily with the next few contractions. A delivery interval of longer than 30 minutes between the first and second twin increases the latter's risk of perinatal mortality and morbidity.
- When cord prolapse or heavy intrapartum bleeding occurs after delivery of the first twin, expeditious breech extraction or, if vertex, application of a Ventouse extractor can bring the head into the pelvis.
- Deliver the placenta by controlled cord traction. Assess carefully the total amount of blood loss and ensure the uterus is well contracted. Delivery of the first placenta before the second twin, if not associated with bleeding, need not cause anxiety.
- Repair the episiotomy, replace blood if necessary and continue with syntocinon if the uterus shows any tendency to relax.
- Examine the placenta for chorionicity.

SURVEILLANCE IN LABOUR

Monitoring the fetal heart rate by scalp electrode for the first twin and by ultrasound for the second twin is the current most satisfactory method of intrapartum surveillance. Fetal blood sampling should be performed to assess signs of distress in the first twin. Clear signs of fetal distress in the second twin necessitate delivery by caesarean section. Deliver by caesarean section if continuous monitoring of the second twin proves difficult.

FURTHER POINTS TO CONSIDER

Box 21.2 lists some further points to consider when delivering twins.

SPECIAL PROBLEMS

Conjoined twins

Suspect this condition when both fetuses are always at the same level and presentation. During labour conjoined twins may present as failure to progress. Radiology or ultrasound scan will help make the diagnosis. Delivery is by use of a midline abdominal incision and classical caesarean section.

Undiagnosed second twin

Oxytocics may have been given before a diagnosis of twin pregnancy is made. The fetus is endangered because of the contracting uterus and the reduced placental blood supply. Proceed as follows:

- Correct the lie and rupture the membranes.
- Forceps/Ventouse for a vertex presentation or a breech extraction is the most expeditious mode of delivery.
- If the fetus is alive and trapped by an undilated cervix deliver by caesarean section.
- If the fetus is dead convert to a longitudinal lie and await vaginal delivery.

Locked twins

This occurs when the head of the first twin delivering as a breech is obstructed by the head

***

Box 21.2 Points to consider in delivery of twins

- Nurse the mother on her side as supine hypotension is more common with the larger uterus.
- Do consider epidural anaesthesia. This will facilitate manipulative delivery for the second twin.
- Ensure anaesthetist, paediatrician and experienced obstetrician are present for the delivery.
- Assess carefully if progress of labour is slow. The total length of labour should not be prolonged. Twin pregnancies enter labour with more cervical dilatation and hence a shorter latent phase; however, the active phase may be lengthened.
- Consider intravenous syntocinon to ensure adequate uterine activity and ensure it is available for use after delivery of the first twin.
- Assess carefully the suitability for vaginal delivery by considering the weaker fetus and the biggest twin.
- Use different clamps on the cords to identify first from second twin.
- Do not miss the diagnosis of twins. Undiagnosed twins impose unnecessary risk for the mother and fetuses.
- Avoid having to perform caesarean section for the second twin after vaginal delivery of the first twin. Proper assessment of suitability for vaginal delivery should obviate this complication. Some 5% of second twins are delivered by caesarean section after vaginal delivery of the first twin. Reasons for this include fetal distress in the second twin, cord prolapse, transverse lie of the second twin or the second twin remaining as a high breech.
- If the second twin is presenting by breech and is much larger than the first twin, deliver by caesarean section. The partially dilated cervix which allowed delivery of the smaller first twin may present difficulty and delay delivery of the larger second breech. A compromise is cephalic version and delivery with a Ventouse extractor.
- If the first twin is presenting by the breech deliver by caesarean section.

***

of the second twin descending into the pelvis. If fetal head cannot be dislodged deliver by classic caesarean section. Decapitation of the first dead twin can be considered. This condition can be avoided if all first twin breeches are delivered by elective caesarean section.

Triplets and higher multiples

The increased risk to the fetus of prematurity, hypoxia and trauma with manipulative delivery supports the use of caesarean section for all deliveries. The placenta covers a large proportion of the uterus, hence placental damage during incision of the uterus is likely with resultant fetal blood loss. Reserve a unit of O negative blood to anticipate need for fetal transfusion. Compared with singleton pregnancies perinatal morbidity and mortality, low birthweight and cerebral palsy rates are much increased.

Antepartum fetal death of one twin

This may occur as in the twin–twin transfusion syndrome. The surviving twin may suffer cerebral and renal lesions and is at risk of intrauterine death. Expect and encourage parents to grieve loss of one of the twins. Parents should know fetal complications may exist before delivery.

FURTHER READING

Adam C, Alexander C A, Vaskett T F 1991 Twin delivery: influence of the presentation and method of delivery on the second twin. American Journal of Obstetrics and Gynecology 165: 23–27

Doherty J 1988 Perinatal mortality in twins, Australia 1973–1980. Acta Geneticae Medicae et Gemellologiae 37: 313–319

Feldman G B 1992 Prospective risk of stillbirth. Obstetrics and Gynaecology 79: 547–553

Fusi C, Gordon H 1990 Twin pregnancy complicated by single intrauterine death: problems and outcome with conservative management. British Journal of Obstetrics and Gynaecology 97: 511–516

Gocke S E, Nageotte M P, Garite T et al 1989 Management of the non-vertex second twin: primary Caesarean section, external version, or primary breech extraction. American Journal of Obstetrics and Gynecology 161: 111–114

Jeffery R L, Watson A, Bowes J R, Delaney J J 1974 Role of bed rest in twin gestation. Obstetrics and Gynaecology 43: 822–826

Kelsick F, Minkoff H 1982 Management of the breech second twin. American Journal of Obstetrics and Gynecology 144: 783–786

Kleinman J C, Fowler M C, Kessel S S 1991 Comparison of infant mortality among twins and singletons; United States 1960–1983. American Journal of Epidemiology 133: 133–143

Little J, Bryan E 1986 Congenital anomalies in twins. Seminars in Perinatology 10(1): 50–64

Newman R B, Hamer C, Millar M C 1989 Outpatient triplet management: a contemporary review. American Journal of Obstetrics and Gynecology 161: 547–555

Petrikovsky B M, Vintzilees A M 1989 Management and outcome of multiple pregnancy of high fetal order: literature review. Obstetrical and Gynecological Survey 44: 578–584

Petterson B, Nelson K B, Watson L, Stanley F 1993 Twins, triplets and cerebral palsy in births in Western Australia in the 1980s. British Medical Journal 307: 1239–1243

Rabinovici J, Barhai G, Reichman B et al 1988 Internal podalic version with unruptured membranes for the second twin in transverse lie. Obstetrics and Gynaecology 71: 428–430

Wolff K 2000 Excessive use of Caesarean section for the second twin? Gynecology, Obstetric Investigation 50: 28–32

22

Medical complications

HAEMATOLOGICAL, COAGULATION, RESPIRATORY AND NEUROLOGICAL DISORDERS

L. Kean

HAEMATOLOGICAL PROBLEMS

Sickle cell disease (HbSS, HbSC, Hb Thal)

- Sickle cell haemoglobin (HbS), a β-chain haemoglobin which affects mothers from Africa, the Middle East, and the Indian sub-continent, can present as persistent anaemia.
- Hypoxia, cold, acidosis, dehydration and infection can precipitate a sickling crisis (see Box 22.1). with resultant tissue infarction and pain. Sickling crisis complicates some 35% of pregnancies. Urinary tract infection, pneumonia and puerperal sepsis are more likely and can cause an acute chest syndrome characterized by fever, tachypnoea, pleuritic chest pain and leucocytosis. Other causes of chest pain include thrombo-embolism and bone marrow embolism.

Box 22.1 Management of sickling crisis

- Enlist haematologist to provide team care.
- Ensure mother is well oxygenated, hydrated and kept warm.
- Provide adequate analgesia.
- Monitor haemoglobin levels. Transfuse if indicated.
- Treat infection.

- Obstetric complications include increased incidence of preterm labour, early onset pre-eclampsia, intrauterine growth retardation and antenatal and intrapartum fetal distress. Maternal and perinatal mortality (increase by 4–6 times) and morbidity are increased.

Labour and delivery

- Keep mother warm, oxygenated (keep oxygen saturation at 97% and monitor by pulse oxymetry) and hydrated (intravenous fluids). Maintain this support for 24 hours post partum.
- Epidural anaesthesia is appropriate.
- Perform caesarean section for obstetric indications.
- Take cord blood for electrophoresis.
- Consider prophylactic antibiotics, for example metronidazole and cephradine, for 7–14 days post partum.
- Administer stockings and heparin (fragmin 5000 units subcutaneously daily) as a prophylaxis for thrombo-embolism even if delivery is vaginal.

Thalassaemia

This condition affects mothers from areas where historically malaria was prevalent, for example South East Asia (thalassaemia α and β), the Middle East, India and the Mediterranean (mainly thalassaemia β). Most mothers are thalassaemia β trait with anaemia as the main risk factor (low mean cell volume (MCV) and mean cell haemoglobin (MCH) with normal mean cell haemoglobin concentration (MCHC)). Diagnosis is by globin chain analysis. Active management of the third stage to limit blood loss is important.

Inherited disorders of coagulation: haemophilia, von Willebrand's disease and factor IX deficiency

von Willebrand's disease (VWD), a result of inherited deficiency in von Willebrand's factor (VWF), affects 0.8–1.3% of mothers. Type I (70% of VWD) mothers produce less VWF with resultant defect of factor VIII. Type II is associated with defective VWF and thrombocytopenia. The rare but severe type III has low levels of both VWF and factor VIII.

Important points

- Haemophilia A (deficiency in factor VIII) with a prevalence of 1 in 10 000 in the population is five times more common than haemophilia B (deficiency in factor IX).
- Inheritance of haemophilia is through sex linkage with carrier mothers having factor VIII or IX levels about 50% of normal.
- Bleeding can occur when levels are below 50% of normal and severity of bleeding is proportional to the degree of deficiency.
- Factor VIII levels tend to rise in pregnancy, as does von Willebrand's factor.

Labour

- Correct low (<50 iu/dl at 36 weeks) levels of factor VIII or IX before labour.
- Notify haematologist when mother is admitted in labour. Site intravenous cannula. Take blood for full blood count, clotting studies and cross-match 4 units of blood.
- Administer relevant blood products in conjunction with haematological advice in any potentially affected fetus.
- Fetal risks include bleeding, cephalohaematoma, subgleal and intracranial haemorrhage. Do not use scalp electrodes or perform fetal blood scalp sampling if the fetus is affected. Ventouse or mid-cavity rotational forceps are contraindicated but a simple lift out is acceptable.
- Avoid prolonged labour or prolonged second stage.
- A low threshold for caesarean section should be considered in prolonged labours.
- Haemostasis is essential when surgery is performed. Repair episiotomy or tears immediately.
- Infuse syntocinon for 4–8 hours after delivery to ensure the uterus remains contracted.
- If shown to be useful before pregnancy, 1-deamino-8-arginine vasopressin (DDAVP) can be helpful for postpartum bleeds in haemophilia A carriers or type I and type IIa VWD.

- Clotting levels may require adjustment over 3–4 days (after vaginal delivery) or 4–5 days (after caesarean section).
- Physiological low levels of factor IX at birth may complicate early diagnosis of haemophilia in the neonate.

Platelet disorders

Platelet disorders are usually due to platelet destruction or consumption, failure of production or splenic sequestration. The commonest problems encountered in pregnancy are due to destruction/consumption, e.g. gestational thrombocytopenia, autoimmune thrombocytopenia.

Causes

- Gestational thrombocytopenia accounts for 70% of this disorder. Normal non-pregnant counts range between 150 and 400×10^9/litre. In gestational thrombocytopenia the counts are usually above 80×10^9/litre and return to normal by 7 days post partum. Diagnosis is by exclusion since aetiology is not known.
- Autoimmune thrombocytopenia (AITP) accounts for 3% of this complication and is often evident before pregnancy. The disorder can be primary (idiopathic) or secondary to systemic lupus erythematosus, antiphospholipid syndromes, drugs, lymphomas plus viral infections, e.g. HIV.
- Non-immune causes include disseminated intravascular coagulation, pre-eclampsia, HELLP (haemolysis elevated liver enzymes low platelets) syndrome, acute fatty liver and heparin induced thrombocytopenia.

Pregnancy

- Take a detailed history and perform clinical examination.
- Examine blood film and instigate other investigations as appropriate.
- A platelet count <20 × 10^9/litre in early pregnancy or <50 × 10^9/litre in late pregnancy requires treatment. In cases of AITP start with prednisolone 30 mg daily for a week. If no response, try intravenous immunoglobulin.

Reserve platelet transfusion for bleeding episodes. In autoimmune thrombocytopenia the risk to the fetus is small. In second pregnancies the best guide of severity is the platelet count of the last baby.

Labour

- Anticipate vaginal delivery unless contra-indicated.
- Elective caesarean section is not necessary purely for thrombocytopenia.
- Epidural anaesthesia is acceptable when the platelet count is above 80×10^9/litre.
- Prescribe prophylactic antibodies if mother had a splenectomy.
- Ensure adequate haemostasis during surgery and prompt repair of episiotomies or tears is mandatory.
- Check cord sample for platelet count.
- Neonatal platelet count is lowest 2–5 days after birth. If count at birth is low, monitor daily until platelet numbers increase. Severe thrombocytopenia requires treatment.

RESPIRATORY PROBLEMS

Respiratory function during labour may be compromised when there is asthma, infection such as pneumonia or tuberculosis (TB), cystic fibrosis or restrictive lung disease.

Asthma

- The most common pre-existing lung condition affecting pregnant women.
- Continue medication during pregnancy.
- Give hydrocortisone 100 mg intravenously in labour (6-hourly until restart of oral medication, if there has been prolonged or recent oral steroid use).
- Epidural anaesthesia is safe. General anaesthesia requires experienced anaesthetist.
- Prostaglandin E_2 is safe. Prostaglandin F_2a is a potent bronchoconstrictor.
- For acute severe attacks in labour (tachypnoea, tachycardia more than 120 beats per minute, severe wheezing and difficulty with speech)

— administer 100% oxygen by mask
— nebulize beta-agonist
— give hydrocortisone 100 mg intravenously.
- Intravenous aminophylline or beta-agonist may be needed in severe attacks.
- Consider ventilatory support if mother is very ill.

Respiratory infections

The fetus is likely to be affected if severe infection causes maternal oxygen saturation to fall below 90% (8 kPa). Infection can precipitate preterm labour. When infection is diagnosed:

- Take blood for full blood count, urea and electrolytes, blood cultures, viral titres and serological test to exclude atypical organisms such as *mycoplasma* or *legionella*.
- Collect sputum for culture and sensitivity and to exclude acidfast bacilli.
- Chest radiology is not contraindicated as there is little risk to the fetus.
- Initiate antibiotics (usually intravenous if infection is severe). Isolation procedures, for example for tuberculosis, may be appropriate. For mothers with tuberculosis the baby should be separated after birth and treated with isoniazid and vaccinated (BCG). If mother is recently treated and cured the baby only requires vaccination.
- An experienced anaesthetist is required if surgical delivery is necessary.

NEUROLOGICAL CONDITIONS

The following are the more usual neurological conditions relevant to labour.

Epilepsy

This condition affects 0.5–1% of childbearing mothers.

- Increased renal and liver clearance of anti-convulsant drugs in pregnancy will lower the pregnancy levels by 10–25%. If fits increase, check drug levels and correct dosage accordingly. Ensure medication is continued during labour.
- Avoid sleep deprivation which results in increased frequency of fits.
- Epileptic mothers have a lower threshold to fit if pre-eclampsia supervenes. Anti-epileptic drugs can potentiate effects of magnesium sulphate. Rule out eclampsia if fits occur during labour.
- Epidural anaesthesia is acceptable.
- Most fits in labour do not need treatment. Lorazepam and diazepam can be used to control fits if prolonged.
- Anticonvulsants decrease maternal (not significant) and fetal vitamin K levels. It is essential to give baby vitamin K after delivery.
- Maternal phenobarbitone can accumulate in baby through breastfeeding.
- Advise mothers against sleep deprivation. Baths should be no more than 3 inches deep. If fits are frequent advise mother to sit on the floor for breastfeeding to avoid dropping baby.

Raised intracranial pressure

This may be benign (benign intracranial hypertension, BIH) or secondary to space-occupying lesions, cerebral oedema, infection, impaired cerebral spinal fluid absorption or drugs.

Management

- Manage secondary raised intracranial pressure with neurologist or neurosurgeon.
- Benign intracranial hypertension is rare but can present for the first time in pregnancy (usually between 8 and 20 weeks). Diagnosis is by exclusion after a normal brain scan and lumbar puncture shows raised intracranial pressure (above 200 mmH_{20}). Presentation includes headaches with or without visual disturbance, bilateral papilloedema and sometimes sixth nerve palsy (inability to abduct eye, with convergent squint and diplopia maximum on lateral gaze to the affected side). Spontaneous resolution in a few months is usual but visual changes can persist. Treatment is to protect visual function.

- Prescribe acetazolamide to reduce cerebrospinal fluid production.
- Repeated lumbar puncture can be performed to drain cerebrospinal fluid.
- Advise weight reduction as condition often occurs in very obese mothers.
- Vaginal delivery with epidural anaesthesia is acceptable. Pushing does not exacerbate the problem.

Neuromuscular disease

Multiple sclerosis, myasthenia gravis and myotonic dystrophy affect mothers of childbearing age with implications in labour.

Multiple sclerosis (MS)

- Pregnancy does not alter course of the disease. Relapse in pregnancy is half that expected but relapse rates are increased post partum. Relapse is also increased after elective termination of pregnancy and is possibly reduced by use of intravenous immunoglobin.
- Manage labour as normal.
- Regional anaesthesia was previously avoided but contemporary lower dose bupivacaine/fentanyl combinations and peridural techniques suggest no increased relapse risk.

Myasthenia gravis

This is an autoimmune disorder of acteylcholine receptors with resultant muscle fatigue, visual disturbance, coughing and speech difficulty. Effect of pregnancy on disease is uncertain. During pregnancy treatment is usually with steroids, anticholinesterase, immunosuppression and plasmaphoresis for life threatening exacerbations. Thymectomy can also be considered if diagnosed before pregnancy.
Management

- Vaginal delivery is safe.
- Administer hydrocortisone 100 mg 6-hourly for 48–72 hours if mother had recent steroid usage.
- Assisted vaginal delivery is usual to overcome muscle fatigue.

- Use regional anaesthesia for caesarean section. Avoid muscle relaxants and opiates. Respiratory function must be carefully monitored postoperatively.
- Magnesium sulphate and gentamicin (neuromuscular blocking properties) are contraindicated.
- Transplacental antibodies cause transient muscle weakness in 20% of neonates. Support is needed for neonatal hypotonia, feeding and respiratory difficulties. Resolution is usually complete by one month.
- Breastfeeding is not contraindicated even if mothers are on steroids or immunosuppressives.

Myotonic dystrophy

This is an autosomal dominant condition with progressive distal muscle weakness, wasting and impaired muscle relaxation leading to loss of facial expression. Frontal balding and cardiovascular complications, which are often evident before 40 years of age, also occur.
Management

- Diagnosis is often made for the first time in early pregnancy. Congenital muscular dystrophy is more common if the mother is affected (rather than the father) as the gene undergoes rapid expansion when passed through the maternal line.
- Perform an electrocardiogram to define cardiovascular status when mothers are admitted to the labour ward if this has not been done.
- Affected fetuses present with polyhydramnios, positional talipes and reduced movement. Preterm labour, stillbirth and neonatal death rates are increased.
- Prescribe syntocinon, as labour is often dysfunctional.
- Assisted vaginal delivery is usual for maternal weakness.
- Regional anaesthesia is the preference for analgesia and for caesarean section. Avoid opiates, which potentiate respiratory compromise. Neuromuscular blockade can be difficult to reverse.
- Postpartum haemorrhage is increased. Infuse syntocinon for 4–8 hours after delivery.

FURTHER READING

Arulkumaran S, Rauff M, Ingemarsson I et al 1986 Uterine activity in myotonia dystrophica. Case report. British Journal of Obstetrics and Gynaecology 93(6): 634–636

Batocchi A P, Majolini L, Evoli A et al 1999 Course and treatment of myasthenia gravis during pregnancy. Neurology 52(3): 447–452

Confavreux C, Hutchinson M, Hours M M et al 1998 Rate of pregnancy-related relapse in multiple sclerosis. Pregnancy in Multiple Sclerosis Group. New England Journal of Medicine 339(5): 285–291

George J N, Woolf S H, Raskob G E et al 1996 Idiopathic thrombocytopenic purpura – a practice guideline developed by explicit methods for the American Society of Hematology. Blood 88: 3–40

Howard R J 1996 Management of sickling conditions in pregnancy. British Journal of Hospital Medicine 56: 7–10

Jaffe R, Mock M, Abramowicz J, Ben-Aderet N 1986 Myotonic dystrophy and pregnancy: a review. Obstetrical and Gynecological Survey 41(5): 272–278

Lusher J M, McMillan C W 1978 Severe factor VIII and factor IX deficiency in females. American Journal of Medicine 65: 637–648

Orvieto R, Achiron R, Rotstein Z et al 1999 Pregnancy and multiple sclerosis: a 2 year experience. European Journal of Obstetrics, Gynecology and Reproductive Biology 82(2): 191–194

Ramsahoye B H, Davies S V, Dasani H et al 1995 Obstetric management in von Willebrand's disease: a report of 24 pregnancies and a review of the literature. Hemophilia 1: 140–144

Weisberg L A 1975 Benign intracranial hypertension. Medicine 54: 197–207

Yerby M S, Freil P N, McCormick K 1992 Antiepileptic drug disposition during pregnancy. Neurology 42 (suppl): 12–16

ENDOCRINE DISORDERS

R. Page

ADRENAL INSUFFICIENCY

Labour and delivery

In response to the stress of labour or surgery the adrenal gland will increase production of corticosteroids. Major stress leads to the secretion of up to 300 mg of cortisol in 24 hours with gradual reduction to usual levels once the stress has been removed. In mothers with adrenal insufficiency additional corticosteroid therapy is required. This should be considered in:

- primary adrenal failure, e.g. Addison's disease
- secondary adrenal failure, e.g. pituitary disease
- previous cortisol therapy – within 1 year
- chronic steroid therapy for other conditions, e.g. asthma.

Various regimens include:

- Hydrocortisone 100 mg (usually sodium succinate) parenterally at the start of labour or with premedication in elective caesarean section. Repeat 8-hourly. In the absence of complications halve the dose daily and switch to oral therapy until maintenance dose is reached.

Fetus

It is unlikely that the short term increase in dosage at the time of delivery will have any effect on the neonate.

THYROID

Hypothyroid

Thyroxine therapy is often increased during pregnancy. No change in thyroxine therapy is required during labour. After birth, reduce thyroxine therapy to pre-pregnancy dose.

Thyrotoxicosis

During pregnancy mothers with thyrotoxicosis should be on the lowest possible dose of propylthiouracil or carbimazole. Propylthiouracil is the preferred therapy. Block and replace therapy should not be used. Maintain thyroid function at the upper end of the normal range. Many mothers become euthyroid and able to discontinue therapy.

Labour and delivery

In well controlled mothers problems are unlikely.

Thyroid storm

This is rare but can occur in a poorly controlled or undiagnosed mother subjected to stress or surgery.

Clinical features include: fever, tachycardia (out of proportion to fever) and other features of thyrotoxicosis, e.g. tremor, restlessness, frequent bowel motions, eye signs.

Management

This is a medical emergency. Follow the procedure below:

- Start treatment whilst waiting for thyroid function assessment to confirm diagnosis.
- Intravenous fluids are needed.
- Give propranolol to block beta-adrenergic reactions and conversion of T4 to T3. Recommended oral doses vary from 160–320 mg/day in divided doses. Intravenous administration should be used if necessary (1–10 mg).
- Propylthiouracil blocks further synthesis of thyroid hormone and T4 to T3 conversion. Give 600 mg orally daily (if necessary via a nasogastric tube). If unavailable use carbimazole.
- Aqueous iodine oral solution (Lugol's iodine) has traditionally been used. Start 1–2 hours after the propylthiouracil. Some now recommend the cholecystographic agents iopanoate or ipodate as, in addition to the iodine which inhibits thyroid secretion, they also block T4 to T3 conversion. One gram is given, followed by a daily dose of 500 mg. However, these agents are not licensed for use in pregnancy and therefore cannot be recommended. Iodides readily cross the placenta and are in breast milk so can cause fetal hypothyroidism and goitre. Use should be limited to thyroid storm.
- Give intravenous hydrocortisone (100 mg 6-hourly) or dexamethasone orally.
- Add supportive therapy – digoxin, oxygen, diuretics and antipyretics as required.

Fetus

Transient neonatal thyrotoxicosis is uncommon. It occurs due to the transplacental passage of maternal immunoglobins. The mother will usually have had a history of thyrotoxicosis but does not have to be hyperthyroid. It is self-limiting but requires treatment as mortality can be high. Maternal thyroid receptor stimulating antibodies can be measured to predict the risk in the neonate. Close intrapartum and postpartum monitoring is required.

DIABETES

All mothers regardless of type of diabetes requiring therapy other than diet during pregnancy will have been treated with insulin. Insulin usage therefore cannot be used to define type of diabetes.

Labour and delivery

Mothers with diabetes are no longer induced early unless for obstetric reasons. However, most obstetricians advise delivery at 39–40 weeks.

Aim to maintain a steady glucose level with neither hypoglycaemia nor hyperglycaemia.

There are many regimens to regulate glucose levels. It is important to become familiar with one to minimize errors in management, e.g. management of mother taking short acting insulin premeal and intermediate at night during labour.

Induction of labour

- The day before induction continue with normal meals and insulin doses.
- On the morning, if prostaglandin pessaries or gel are to be used and it is thought labour will be slow to proceed, normal meals and insulin should be given (usually breakfast and morning dose of insulin).
- Measure blood glucose hourly in active labour.
- At artificial rupture of membranes/spontaneous rupture of membranes control glucose by glucose infusion at a constant rate and insulin

at a variable rate to maintain a normal blood glucose (4–7 mmol/l).

— Infuse 5% glucose at a rate of 100 ml/hour controlled by an infusion pump (5 g glucose every hour).

— Make up 50 units of short acting soluble insulin (e.g. Actrapid) to a volume of 50 cc with normal saline in a 50 cc syringe, to be infused by pump (one unit of insulin per ml).

— Monitor blood glucose half hourly to hourly. It is advisable to send a venous sample to the laboratory at the start of labour to double check the accuracy of the meter being used.

— Adjust infusion rate of insulin according to blood glucose measurements. One to two units of insulin per hour are usually required.

— Test all urine samples for ketones.

— Check electrolytes. It may be necessary to add potassium to the infusion.

— Encourage use of epidural anaesthesia for pain and metabolic control.

— If it is required, infuse syntocinon in normal saline not glucose.

Spontaneous labour

Check food intake and insulin usage. Test for ketones. Manage as for induction of labour (see Table 22.1). If blood sugar levels are high omit glucose until control achieved.

Caesarean section

In consultation with anaesthetist start infusion of glucose/insulin before anaesthesia and continue in theatre. Elective caesarean sections are ideally performed in the morning. Ensure blood sugar levels are between 5.0 and 7.0 mmol/l before surgery.

After delivery continue glucose insulin infusion overnight with regular, e.g. 2-hourly, blood glucose monitoring. Due to decreased insulin requirements a change to 10% glucose and/or decrease in insulin infusion rate may be required. Discontinue infusion and return to pre-pregnancy

Table 22.1 Guide for insulin infusion with 30 minutes blood sugar monitoring

Blood glucose (mmol/l)	Insulin infusion (ml/hour)
Below 4.0	Stop insulin. Check infusion system. Consider oral or parenteral glucose (10% dextrose)
4.0–6.0	1 unit of insulin/hour
6.0–8.0	2 units of insulin/hour
Above 8.0	3 units of insulin/hour
More than 12.0	3 units of insulin/hour. Stop glucose

insulin dose when mother is eating and drinking. Continue 4-hourly blood glucose monitoring.

Management of mothers not requiring insulin

Take hourly blood tests. Consider starting infusion of glucose and insulin when blood glucose rises above 7 mmol/l.

It should be remembered that the following are more common:

- large for dates babies
- assisted delivery
- fetal hypoglycaemia
- congenital abnormality in offspring of pre-existing diabetic mothers.

Post delivery

- Gestational diabetes: stop insulin and monitor blood glucose twice daily for a few days. At 6 weeks after birth perform glucose tolerance test. Remember, although uncommon, mothers may have had newly diagnosed Type I diabetes.

- Type II diabetes: return to previous pre-pregnancy therapy. Oral hypoglycaemics are not recommended for breastfeeding mothers. If therapy is required insulin can be used, often at a greatly reduced dosage from that during pregnancy.

- Type I diabetes: after delivery insulin requirements return to pre-pregnancy levels. Decrease glucose/insulin infusion rate. Once eating use pre-pregnancy insulin doses. Further dosage reduction may be required:

— during the first 24 hours
— if breastfeeding
— when pre-pregnancy control was very tight.
- After normal delivery:
  — for delivery before midday give quick acting insulin with lunch and normal regimen before evening meal
  — for delivery after evening meal give medium acting insulin that night and normal pre-pregnancy regimen next day.

Fetus

Complications, especially hypoglycaemia, are more common. Close monitoring of blood sugar is required.

Medical emergencies

Diabetic ketoacidosis and hypoglycaemic coma should be treated along conventional lines.

FURTHER READING

British National Formulary 1999 Section 6 Endocrine system, vol 38. BMJ Books, British Medical Association, London

Burger A G, Philippe J 1992 Thyroid emergencies. In: Burger A G, Philippe J (eds) Clinical endocrinology and metabolism. Baillière Tindall, London, vol 6, no. 1, p 77–93

Livanou T, Ferriman D, James V H T 1967 Recovery of hypothalamo-pituitary adrenal function after corticosteroid therapy. Lancet 2: 856–859

Pregnancy and Neonatal Group 1996 Saint Vincent and improving diabetes care specialist UK (workgroup reports). Diabetic Medicine Supplement 13(4): S43–S53

CARDIAC DISEASE

P. Baker

Common disorders include rheumatic heart disease (with or without prosthetic heart valves), congenital anomalies (for example the tetralogy of Fallot, Eisenmenger's syndrome) and cardiomyopathies of varying severity. The incidence of congenital heart disease in pregnancy is increasing because mothers with more severe defects can have corrective surgery as children and are now able to have children themselves.

Mothers with cardiac disease or defects are at risk of:

- Pulmonary oedema (precipitated by anxiety, pain, exertion, infection and tachycardia) when there is obstruction to cardiac outflow, as in mitral or aortic stenosis.
- Cardiac syncopy and cyanosis. This follows hypertension, excessive blood loss, or any cause of poor venous return in mothers with defects such as the tetralogy of Fallot.
- Bacterial endocarditis. This infection is usually associated with *Streptococcus* (principally *viridans* and *faecalis*), *Staphylococcus* (*albus* and *aureus*) or gram negative organisms. Prevention by prophylactic antibiotics is essential.
- Arrhythmia.

LABOUR

- With the onset of labour or 1–2 hours before elective caesarean section, give amoxycillin 1 g intravenous/intramuscular and gentamicin (120 mg intravenous/intramuscular). When penicillin allergy is present, use vancomycin 1 g intravenously, or teicoplanin 400 mg intravenously.
- Ensure comfortable labour, avoid hypotension.
- Use the semirecumbent or lateral position. The supine and especially the lithotomy position should be avoided as much as possible to minimize the risk of pulmonary oedema.
- Apply continuous ECG and monitor oxygen saturation. Full resuscitation facilities must be available.
- Beware of vasodilatation and hypotension with epidural blocks in mothers with limited stroke volume and left ventricular outlet flow obstruction (e.g. aortic stenosis, hypertrophic cardiomyopathy (HOCM)).

- If a pudendal block is required, lidocaine (lignocaine) without adrenaline should be used.

DELIVERY

There should be a low threshold for assisted delivery if birth is not achieved within 20 minutes after onset of second stage. Reserve caesarean section for the usual indications. Avoid ergometrine, give syntocinon 10 units intramuscularly and by subsequent intravenous infusion to control post-partum bleeding. All mothers must be observed carefully for at least 24 hours after delivery. Transfer to a high dependency or intensive care unit may be appropriate.

FETUS

The fetus suffers as a consequence of maternal hypoxia and hypotension. Continuous fetal heart rate monitoring should be employed throughout labour.

MYOCARDIAL INFARCTION

Box 22.2 lists points to note in cases of myocardial infarction at term.

ACUTE PULMONARY OEDEMA

The mother experiences acute dyspnoea with frothy sputum. Characteristic moist sounds are audible at the lung bases. Hypoxaemia and increased lung vascular markings are present.

Confirm diagnosis

Chest X-ray, pulse oximetry and arterial blood gases (acute acidosis with consequent decreased pH and increased PCO_2 but only slight alteration in base excess).

Management

- Involve cardiologist to provide team care.
- Provide supportive measures. These include oxygen administration via facemask and

---

Box 22.2 Myocardial infarction at term

- Rare but will present more frequently as older mothers and those with pre-existing heart disorders are becoming pregnant.
- Incidence of 1 in 10000 maternities with 45% maternal mortality and 34% fetal loss.
- Presents with classic symptoms of chest tightness, pain and shortness of breath. Aetiology is usually structural pathology or coronary artery thrombosis with a transmural rather than subendo-cardial infarct.
- Occurrence is usually during labour or immediately following delivery.
- Team care with cardiologist and anaesthetist is mandatory.
- Maternal mortality rate is higher if delivery is within 2 weeks of an acute myocardial infarct.
- Cardiac output increases 50% in the second stage of labour. Each contraction pushes 300–500 ml of blood into the general circulation causing increase in stroke volume, cardiac output (up by 15%) and increased arterial pressure. Vaginal delivery, if appropriate, necessitates:
  — electrocardiographic monitoring (ECG)
  — epidural analgesia (pain increases release of catecholamines)
  — elective assisted instrumental vaginal delivery
  — cardiotocograph monitoring of the fetus
  — avoid ergometrine; oxytocin reduces coronary blood flow and levels above that used for labour induction or control of post-partum atony may not be safe.
- Elective caesarean section is the preferred mode of delivery but cardiac output still increases by 50%.

---

nursing with head elevation above the level of the right atrium. Measure oxygen saturation of the circulating blood via pulse oximetry.
- Maintain fluid balance by careful monitoring of intake and output. Serum electrolytes must be closely monitored especially in mothers receiving diuretics. The use of a pulmonary artery catheter will help distinguish between fluid overload, left ventricular dysfunction and pulmonary oedema associated with vascular bed injury.
- Perform frequent arterial blood gas measurements to assess the underlying respiratory status.
- Administer furosemide (frusemide) (10–40 mg) intravenously over 1–2 minutes. Larger doses may be required if diuresis does not ensue.
- If left ventricular failure is suspected, reduction in preload by agents such as glycerol trinitrate

may help. Likewise, hydralazine may be employed to reduce the after load.

- Treat arrhythmia if present (paroxysmal supraventricular tachycardia and atrial fibrillation are more common in pregnancy).
- Involve an anaesthetist; hypoxia may persist despite treatment and mechanical ventilation may be required.

HYPERTENSION

This is diagnosed where a blood pressure (BP) of 140/90 mmHg or more is recorded on two separate occasions at least 6 hours apart. Causes include chronic hypertension, chronic renal disease, endocrine disorders (phaeochromocytoma) and coarctation of the aorta, in addition to pregnancy induced hypertension (mothers are normotensive prior to 20th week of pregnancy). If presenting in labour:

- Check blood pressure at 15 minute intervals to confirm diagnosis.
- Test urine for protein.
- Engage care team when diagnosis is made.

PRE-ECLAMPSIA

Pre-eclampsia is defined as confirmed BP of ≥140/90 mmHg, proteinuria 2 pluses, or more than 300 mg urinary protein in 24 hours.

This multi-systemic disorder of pre-eclampsia is pregnancy induced hypertension with the addition of significant proteinuria. In pregnancy, protein excretion may be considerably increased but up to 300 mg of total protein per 24 hours is accepted as normal. A 24 hour measurement of urinary protein should confirm the diagnosis. When this is not possible, alternative approaches include setting a high limit for diagnosis such as 2 pluses protein on dipstick testing or a concentration of 1 g protein/litre in a random sample.

Management of pre-eclampsia: investigation and assessment

- Obtain detailed obstetric history and perform clinical examination. Both mother and fetus are affected by this condition. Carry out neurological examination noting the presence or absence of hyperreflexia, clonus (more than 3 beats), focal neurological defects and papilloedema. On abdominal examination, epigastric tenderness and hepatic tenderness indicate subcapsular liver haemorrhages. Note non-dependent oedema.
- Haematological: take blood for group and save, platelet count, clotting screen and biochemical tests.
- Biochemical: check urea and electrolytes. An elevated plasma uric acid is used as an indicator of impaired renal function and renal blood flow. (Note other conditions which increase plasma uric acid.) Abnormal liver function tests (increase in lactate dehydrogenase and transaminase) relate to altered liver perfusion or hepatic congestion. Note HELLP syndrome.
- General care includes obstetric assessment, ultrasound scan if appropriate, continuous heart rate monitoring, regular pulse and BP check (every 15 minutes), and monitor hourly urinary output with an indwelling catheter. Adjust degree of surveillance to severity of pre-eclampsia.

Antihypertensive therapy

Aim is to protect the mother by minimizing the risks of cerebral haemorrhage, cardiac failure or myocardial infarct and placental abruption. Although there is no specific threshold for such events, the risks are significant when the blood pressure exceeds 170/110 mmHg. Commence treatment at this level. Treatment does not prevent disease progression – there is no place for complacency. Treatment must induce a smooth sustained fall in blood pressure. Hydralazine and labetalol are drugs which can fulfil this requirement. Typical regimens are: hydralazine, bolus 5–10 mg intravenously followed by 10 mg per hour (max 40 mg per hour), doubling every 30 minutes until a satisfactory response is achieved (diastolic blood pressure 90 mmHg ±5 mmHg); or labetalol, bolus 20 mg intravenously followed by infusion of 40 mg per hour (max 60 mg per

---

Box 22.3 Management of hypertensive crisis

- Defined as blood pressure of 170/110 mmHg or more.
- Give intravenously hydralazine 5–10 mg in 10 ml of normal saline over 10 minutes. Monitor BP every 5 minutes until level is between 140/80 and 160/100 mmHg. Note BP may drop 20 minutes after this bolus dose.
- Use 50 mg hydralazine in 50 ml normal saline to give 1 mg/ml and deliver by syringe pump for subsequent control of hypertension. Note side effects which include tachycardia, hot flushes, facial erythema, headaches.
- Labetalol (see above) is an alternative therapy.

Editor's note: ketanserin 20 mg bolus over 1 minute and repeat with 5–10 mg in 10 minutes followed by infusion of 2–14 mg/hour has also been prescribed in some European centres.

---

hour), doubling every 30 minutes until satisfactory response is achieved.

Box 22.3 gives guidance for managing a hypertensive crisis.

Anticonvulsant therapy

Magnesium sulphate ($MgSo_4$) reduces the incidence of recurrent convulsions after an eclamptic fit. Prophylactic treatment in pre-eclampsia reduces the number of fits and improves maternal outcome.

Procedure

- Magnesium sulphate is dispensed as 50% w/v solution with 1 g in 2 ml.
- Suggested regimen is 4 g loading dose (8 ml 50% w/v $MgSo_4$ in 20 ml 5% dextrose) intravenously over 20 minutes, then maintenance dose of 2 g per hour (monitor serum levels). The infusion should be continued for 24 hours after delivery or until a maternal diuresis (>100 ml of urine for 2 consecutive hours) has commenced. For fits during infusion add 2 mg $MgSo_4$ intravenously over 2–3 minutes if drug levels are low.
- Contraindications include cardiac disease (digoxin therapy). In renal failure (less than 30 ml urine per hour over 2 hours) use with extreme caution. $MgSo_4$ will potentiate neuromuscular blocking agents.
- Monitor by clinical observations (deep tendon reflexes, ECG/pulse oximetry) and by plasma levels (therapeutic range 2–3 mmol/l). At 4–5.5 mmol/l there is loss of patella reflex, weakness, nausea, flushing, double vision, slurred speech, hypotension and hypothermia. At 6–7.5 mmol/l the mother experiences muscle paralysis and respiratory arrest. At >12 mmol/l there is cardiac arrest.
- Fetal side effects include flaccidity, hyporeflexia and respiratory depression.
- Hypermagnesaemia in mother also results in flushing, sweating, hypotension, depressed reflexes, cardiac, respiratory and neurological function, hypothermia, flaccid paralysis and collapse.
- The antidote is 10–20 ml of 10% calcium gluconate intravenously.

Fluid balance

- Hypovolaemia associated with pre-eclampsia necessitates close attention to fluid balance to protect the kidneys and prevent pulmonary oedema.
- Urine output is best monitored by siting an indwelling urethral catheter and taking measurements hourly.
- Fluid input should be no more than 1 ml per kilogram per hour (normal saline is the fluid of choice).
- Delivery quickly reverses the effects of pre-eclampsia on renal function. If not, invasive monitoring with central venous pressure (CVP) lines, or more accurately by pulmonary capillary wedge pressure readings, should be considered.

General management

- Involve haematologist for multidisciplinary management if there is evidence of coagulopathy.
- There are few contraindications to use of epidural anaesthesia. Thrombocytopenia

(platelet count $<50 \times 10^9/l$) is an absolute contraindication.

- Delivery is mandatory when pre-eclampsia is diagnosed at term. The dilemma occurs in mothers with early onset of pre-eclampsia between 24 and 34 weeks gestation. If the severity of the disease necessitates antihypertensive and anticonvulsant therapy as detailed above, deliver once the mother's condition is stabilized. Mode of delivery depends upon the gestational age and severity of disease.
- The fetus is at risk of hypoxia if there is associated growth restriction or placental insufficiency. Close intrapartum surveillance is mandatory.
- Second stage should be short. Assisted instrumental delivery is recommended for delay (more than 30 minutes).
- Ergometrine should be avoided in the third stage as it may precipitate eclampsia – syntocinon 10 units should be administered.
- Observe mother closely for 24 hours after delivery.

ECLAMPSIA

Eclampsia (*flashing lights*) is the occurrence of convulsions, not attributable to other cerebral causes, in association with the signs and symptoms of pre-eclampsia. The risk of eclampsia is low (1%) even if there is severe pre-eclampsia.

The initial eclamptic fit should be controlled by either an intravenous bolus of 4 mg of magnesium sulphate over 20 minutes or an intravenous bolus of diazepam (10 mg intravenously over 1 minute). Thereafter a magnesium sulphate infusion should be commenced.

RENAL FAILURE

Renal failure is a rare complication of pre-eclampsia and usually follows acute blood loss, when there has been inadequate transfusion, or after profound hypotension. Oliguria without rising urea or creatinine is a manifestation of severe pre-eclampsia and not of incipient renal failure.

Procedure

- Oliguria (<400 ml/24 hours) is not an indication for treatment if mothers are well perfused.
- Loop diuretic furosemide (frusemide) or osmotic diuretic (mannitol) administration temporarily improves urine output but further decreases circulating blood volume and disturbs electrolyte balance.
- Consult a renal physician if renal failure is suspected.
- Without invasive monitoring, repetitive fluid challenges should be avoided.
- If there is no response to therapeutic measures suspect occurrence of acute corticol necrosis.

FURTHER READING

Chua S, Redman C W 1991 Are prophylactic anticonvulsants required in severe pre-eclampsia? Lancet 337: 250–251

Duley L, Gulmezoglu A M, Henderson-Smart D 1999 Anticonvulsants for women with pre-eclampsia. In Cochrane Collaboration. Cochrane Library, Issue 1, Update Software, Oxford

Gulmezoglu M, Duley L 1998 Use of anticonvulsants in eclampsia and pre-eclampsia: survey of obstetricians in the United Kingdom and the Republic of Ireland. British Medical Journal 316: 975–976

Hayman R G, Baker P N 2000 Labour ward management of pre-eclampsia. In: Kean L H, Baker P N, Edlestone D I (eds) Best practice in labour ward management. W B Saunders, Edinburgh, p 253–294

Lipsite P J 1971 The clinical and biochemical effects of excess magnesium in the newborn. Paediatrics 47: 501–509

The Eclamptic Trial Collaborative Group 1995 Which anticonvulsant for women with eclampsia? Evidence from the collaborative eclampsia trial. Lancet 345: 1455–1463

Tucker D, Liu D T Y, Ramoutar O 1996 Myocardial infarction at term: a case report to consider management options. Journal of Obstetrics and Gynaecology 16: 52–54

INFECTIONS

C. Bowman

BACTERIAL

Amniotic fluid may become infected. Mothers with diabetes, prolonged membrane rupture or repeated catheterization of the bladder are more prone to infection.

Maternal signs

Pyrexia (the temperature may be normal or subnormal with gram negative infections) and tachycardia are usual.

Fetal signs

Persistent tachycardia and evidence of fetal distress (fetal heart rate pattern changes and fetal acidosis) are present.

Bacteraemia and septic shock

Organisms include *Escherichia coli,* other gram negative bacilli, *Staphylococcus aureus,* anaerobic infections including *Bacteroides* spp, Group B streptococcus, *Listeria monocytogenes.*

Symptoms are high fever (temperature may be low or normal in gram negative septicaemia), nausea, vomiting, malaise, tachycardia (sometimes). There are symptoms from the infection source e.g. dysuria.

Septic shock

This is characterized by profound hypotension, cold clammy skin, tachycardia, tachypnoea, oliguria.

Management

- Collect two sets of blood cultures.
- Urine for microscopy and culture (other samples as indicated, e.g. CSF if signs of meningism).

- Administer broad spectrum antibiotics intravenously chosen on the basis of likely source, local antibiotic resistance patterns and severity of illness, e.g. ampicillin, gentamicin and metronidazole or cefotaxime plus metronidazole.
- Give appropriate loading doses and monitor gentamicin levels subsequently.
- Consult on-call microbiologist for advice.
- Give treatment for shock including careful fluid maintenance, electrolyte balance, blood sugar monitoring. If severe may require immediate admission to intensive care.

Labour and delivery

- Locate the cause of infection.
- Maternal infection can interfere with uterine activity.
- Fetal infection results in fetal tachycardia and early onset of fetal distress. Consider a caesarean section if delivery is not expected in 1–2 hours or if fetal distress is evident.
- Obtain blood, urine and amniotic fluid for culture. Administer antibiotics as described.
- An experienced paediatrician should attend the delivery.
- Obtain samples from the placenta for culture.
- Take samples for bacteriological screening of the neonate.

Group B haemolytic streptococcus (GBS)

This is a major cause of maternal bacteraemia, premature labour, postpartum endometritis and neonatal bacteraemia and meningitis.

GBS is a normal commensal of the vagina or intestinal tract in 15–30% of women. Mothers can be chronic, transient or intermittent carriers. Some 40–73% of babies are colonized but only 1–2% develop disease within 7 days after vaginal delivery. In 80% disease onset is within 48 hours. Mortality rate of infected babies is 10–20%.

Positive culture is most likely from the rectum and vaginal swabs. Note 50% of carriers can be missed. A positive urinary culture sometimes indicates vaginal colonization.

Management

- Population screening is of little value.
- Mothers at risk include:
  - previous infected baby (10 times increased risk)
  - mothers with positive cultures (4 times increased risk if GBS detected in urine or recto-vaginal area)
  - positive culture and preterm labour (before 37 weeks)
  - ruptured membranes of more than 18 hours (prescribe intravenous antibiotics for 24 hours followed by treatment for 10 days or until delivery; repeat swabs and continue treatment if GBS persists)
  - intrapartum pyrexia of 38°C or more and evidence of infection (tender uterus or fetal tachycardia).
- Antibiotic therapy includes:
  - intravenous loading dose of penicillin, e.g. 2.4 g intravenous benzylpenicillin or ampicillin (2 g) followed by 4–6-hourly doses as appropriate until delivery
  - use clindamycin (600 mg intravenously 6-hourly) or erythromycin (500 mg intravenously 6-hourly) if allergic to penicillin
  - note 10% of mothers will have a mild allergic reaction to penicillin, 1 in 1000 will develop anaphylaxis and this anaphylaxis proves fatal in 1 in 100 000 of those affected.

Listerosis (*listeria monocytogenes*)

This organism gains access to the amniotic cavity through haematogenous spread and may cause bacteraemia, preterm labour, severe sepsis, meningoencephalitis and fetal death. Infection is usually acquired by eating pâté and unpasteurized milk products.

Maternal symptoms

- Fever
- Headaches
- Myalgia
- Flu-like symptoms
- Evidence of chorioamnionitis.

Diagnosis

- Blood cultures from mother and neonate
- Neonate CSF, tracheal/gastric aspirates; meconium specimens.

Management

- High dose intravenous ampicillin plus gentamicin.

Chlamydia trachomatis

- Endocervical infection is common in 15–25 year olds (10–15%).
- Genital infection in the mother may be asymptomatic.
- Vertical transmission in labour may cause conjunctivitis, pneumonia and otitis media.
- Postpartum complication includes pelvic inflammatory disease, endometritis and cervicitis.

Diagnosis

Depends on local laboratory. This includes enzyme immunoassays (EIA), test or culture from endocervical swab and ligase chain reaction (LCR) or polymerase chain reaction (PCR) test on urine or vaginal swab. In about 20% of infected mothers gonorrhoea is also present.

Management

- Treat mother with erythromycin or azithromycin (amoxyl may be used if mother is intolerant of erythromycin).
- Neonatal infection requires systemic erythromycin.
- Refer mother to Department of Genitourinary Medicine for follow-up and contact tracing. Fifty per cent of babies with infected mothers develop conjunctivitis. Babies need oral erythromycin.

VIRAL

Genital herpes (HSV)

- May be caused by either *Herpes simplex* type I or II (incubation period 2–7 days).

- Mothers who acquire genital herpes during pregnancy have a significant risk of vertical transmission to their babies. Some 5% of neonatal infections are intrauterine following transplacental or ascending transmembrane spread.
- The risk of neonatal herpes is extremely low if the mother acquired her genital herpes before conception. The risk is 40–50% with primary but less than 5% with recurrent infection.

Diagnosis

- 75% of *Herpes simplex* infections in mothers are asymptomatic hence there is no warning history in 60% of neonatal infections.
- Clinical appearance (confirm with culture). Mothers may experience burning or pain. Vesicles, ulcers and lymphadenopathy are present.
- Culture of HSV from an herpetic ulcer.

Management

- Examine vulva and cervix for ulcers.
- Deliver fetus by caesarean section if active infection during labour. This is advised even if membranes have ruptured more than 6 hours.
- For mothers who develop their first episode of genital herpes in the third trimester of pregnancy, delivery should be by caesarean section. If vaginal delivery is unavoidable, acyclovir should be given to the mother and baby to prevent vertical transmission. Acyclovir, however, may not prevent viral shedding.

Chronic bloodborne viruses

General measures

- Prevention of nosocomial infection by standard infection control procedures, e.g. safe disposal of sharps, use of disposable items where possible (e.g. plastic speculae), decontamination of spillages, etc.
- Prevention of occupational infection:
  — appropriate use of gloves, eye protection, gowns, covering of minor cuts/abrasions
  — vaccination for hepatitis B

  — follow local post-exposure prophylaxis guidelines if needlestick injury occurs.

Identify mothers at risk of human immunodeficiency viral infection and viral hepatitis by sensitive history taking and implementation of new guidelines on antenatal testing.

Hepatitis B (HB)

- Caused by a hepatitis B virus (HBV). Incubation period 50–180 days.
- Virus is present in all body secretions and fluid. Infection results in neonatal morbidity and mortality.
- Infectivity and risk of vertical transmission depend on both HBsAg and eAg status. HBsAg and e antigen positive mothers are most infectious. Ten per cent vertical transmission if mother only positive for HBsAg – 90% if both HBsAg and HBeAg positive.
- Deliver according to usual obstetric indications.
- Following delivery baby should be vaccinated for hepatitis B and given hepatitis B immunoglobulin in the other thigh if the mother is either eAg positive or lacking any 'e' markers (babies of mothers with antibody to HBe are given vaccine only).

Hepatitis C

- Prevalence of 1–2% in mothers. Transfusion and drug abuse are risk factors.
- Vertical transmission can occur but risks are much less than for hepatitis B (2–5%).
- No vaccine or passive immunoglobulin currently available.
- Avoid interventions which breach fetal skin e.g. scalp electrodes.
- Breastfeeding is controversial.

Human immunodeficiency virus (HIV)

- Virus is present in all body fluids. Antibodies appear 3–6 months after initial infection. Maternal viral load is important.
- The risk of vertical transmission can be reduced from 15–40% to 2% by the appropriate use of

antiretroviral drugs and caesarean section. In utero infection can occur.

- Zidovudine (antiretroviral therapy) alone can reduce transmission (by more than 60%) to 5–8% of neonatal infection. If not treated previously administer zidovudine 2 mg/kg body weight intravenously over 1 hour then 1 mg/kg body weight hourly until cord clamped.
- Pregnancy, labour and neonatal care should be carefully managed by close liaison between obstetrician, HIV physician and neonatologist.
- If the mother is on anti-HIV drugs these should be continued during labour and post partum. The mother's HIV physician will advise on the need for additional zidovudine during labour.
- The neonate should receive zidovudine syrup 2 mg/kg every 6 hours starting within 12 hours of delivery. Zidovudine is continued for 6 weeks in the neonate. Septrin prophylaxis is started at 3 weeks.
- Delivery by elective caesarean section is recommended. Intravenous zidovudine should be started 3 hours before surgery and continue until the cord is clamped.
- Breastfeeding should be avoided in developed countries.
- Combination of antiretroviral therapy, caesarean section and avoidance of breastfeeding reduce vertical transmission to less than 2%.

Varicella zoster (Chicken pox)

- Incubation period 10–24 days. Infectious 48 hours before rash until crusting of vesicles.
- 85–90% of mothers are sero positive. Primary attack with maternal pneumonitis (10%) is associated with 1% mortality rates. Risk of pneumonia increases in later gestation.
- Babies born within 7–28 days of delivery to mothers with chicken pox can develop neonatal varicella with a 20–30% mortality. Severe neonatal infection is most likely if baby is born within 7 days of onset of mother's rash. Administer 250 mg zoster immune globulin. Consider prophylactic acyclovir.
- Does not cause miscarriage but fetal varicella syndrome (eye problems, limb hypoplasia, microencephaly, mental retardation, bowel and bladder sphincter dysfunction) complicates 1–2% if mother is infected before 20 weeks of pregnancy. Viral complication is unlikely after 20 weeks of pregnancy.
- Immunoglobin is effective up to 10 days after contact. If mother is not sure of immunity and was in contact, check immunity status before giving immunoglobins.
- At the viraemic phase the mother is at risk of bleeding, thrombocytopenia, disseminated intravascular coagulopathy and hepatitis.

FURTHER READING

Dillon H C, Khare S, Gray B M 1987 Group b streptococcal carriage and disease: a 6 year prospective study. Journal of Paediatrics 110: 31–36

Kenyon S L, Taylor D J, Tarnow-Mordi W 2001 Broad spectrum antibiotics for spontaneous preterm labour: the Oracle II randomised trial. Lancet 357: 989–994

Kim K S 1985 Antimicrobial susceptibility of GBS. Antibiotics and Chemotherapy 35: 83–89

O'Reilly G C, Hitti J E, Benedetti T J 1999 Group b streptococcus infection in pregnancy: an update. Fetal and Maternal Medicine Review 11: 31–39

Siegel J D 1998 Prophylaxis for neonatal Group b streptococcus infection. Seminar of Perinatology 22: 33–49

Taylor G P, Hermione Lyall E G, Mercey D et al 1999 British HIV Association guideline for prescribing antiretroviral therapy in pregnancy (1998). Sexually Transmitted Infections 75: 90–97

Royal College of Obstetricians and Gynaecologists 2001 Guideline number 13. Chickenpox in pregnancy. RCOG Press, London 1–8

PSYCHIATRIC ILLNESS

D. Liu

GENERAL POINTS

- 10–20% of newly delivered mothers will develop a depressive illness with 3–5% of them being severely depressed (2 per 1000). Suicide ranks high although it is not the most common cause of maternal death in the year following delivery. Some 1–2 per 1000 mothers develop a psychotic illness after delivery.
- 2 per 1000 mothers will suffer a relapse of their pre-existing psychotic and affective disorders.
- At-risk mothers include those with
  - a personal or close family history of affective disorder, severe depression or puerperal psychosis
  - panic disorder, severe anxiety or schizophrenia.
- After delivery watch out for obsessive or psychotic symptoms, severe anxiety, expression of guilt, suicidal intent and feelings of unworthiness.

DRUG MISUSER

- There is no typical misuser and non-disclosure is common because of fear that lifestyle will be scrutinized or that baby may be taken away into care.
- Drug users encounter a high incidence of preterm labour, fetal growth retardation, intrauterine fetal death and cot deaths. Close fetal monitoring in labour is essential.
- Do not withdraw drugs suddenly.
- Watch out for infections such as bacterial endocarditis, hepatitis B and C or HIV.
- Encourage contact between mother and baby to maximize bonding.
- Protect confidentiality of the mother as a drug user. Her relatives may not be aware of her habits.

Opiate user

- Treat as if infection may be present.
- Opiate receptors are saturated hence these mothers will need large doses of drugs for analgesia. Do not use opiates if the mother is weaned from her habit. Epidural anaesthesia for pain relief is recommended.
- Risk of placental insufficiency is increased. Avoid use of fetal scalp clips. Continuous external cardiotocographic monitoring for the fetus is essential but note opiates can interfere with interpretation of fetal heart rate patterns.
- There is no evidence of long term organ damage in the baby.
- Do not give Narcan to baby after baby is born if mother has been using opiates.
- Withdrawal symptoms start in the baby within 24–48 hours after delivery. There is usually a high pitched cry, tachycardia, restlessness, sweating, fever, vomiting, diarrhoea or fits.

Cocaine user

- This vasoconstrictor can cause maternal hypertension, tachycardia and placental abruption. The hypertension can confuse diagnosis of pre-eclampsia.
- Levels of protein C and antithrombin III are reduced, hence an increased risk of thrombosis. On the other hand thrombocytopenia may be encountered so platelets must be checked before insertion of epidural anaesthesia.
- Monitor fetus during labour as placental insufficiency and fetal growth retardation are likely.
- Use phenylephrine or methoxamine for treatment of hypotension associated with epidural usage.

User of benzodiazepines, for example temazepam or diazepam

- There is increased risk of cleft palate.
- Babies with withdrawal symptoms may have low temperatures, poor muscle tone with poor sucking and respiratory difficulties.
- Breastfeeding is not recommended.

Amphetamine user

- Mothers may be malnourished and complain of tiredness.
- Intrauterine growth retardation is common.

Cannabis user

- No specific harmful side effects for mother.
- Intrauterine growth retardation is common.

REFERENCES

Cox J L, Murray P, Chapman E 1993 A controlled study of the onset, duration and prevalence of postnatal depression. British Journal of Psychiatry 163: 27–31

DoH 1998 Confidential enquiry into maternal deaths in the UK. Why mothers die (1994–1996). HMSO, London

English National Board 1997 Substance misuse – guidelines for good practice. ENB, London

Kendell R E, Chalmers J C, Platz C 1987 Epidemiology of puerperal psychosis. British Journal of Psychiatry 150: 662–672

Royal College of Psychiatrists 2000 Recommendations for the provision of mental health services for child bearing women. Royal College of Psychiatrists, London

23

Fetal and maternal misadventure

D. Liu, C. Rodeck

It is a sad but undeniable fact that, despite the best intentions, fetal and maternal damage or death occasionally complicate labour. The maternal mortality rate in England and Wales is around 1 per 10 000 live births (see Ch. 3). This can mean a tragedy about every 2 years in an obstetric department subserving 5000 pregnancies annually. The corrected perinatal mortality of around 1 per 100 births is 100 times higher than the maternal mortality rate. When misfortune presents itself appropriate counselling is essential. In most units a risk management form must be completed.

FETAL ABNORMALITIES

- The mother and her partner should be informed at the earliest opportunity of any major abnormality found at birth. Minor defects that are detected can be discussed later, at an appropriate time. Monstrosities are best not shown to parents unless explicitly requested and only after sensitive preparation.
- Discuss fully the likely cause and consequence of the abnormality. If appropriate arrange paediatric and genetic counselling for the couple.
- 3% of births are associated with an abnormality of some sort. Parents naturally want to identify a possible cause. Discuss all queries or suggestions and discourage any feelings of guilt.
- Rejection of the abnormal baby is a natural first reaction. Frequent discussion and counselling in the postnatal period is essential.
- All congenital abnormalities incompatible with life should be photographed, X-rayed and

karyotyped to enhance subsequent genetic counselling.

- In contemporary practice most abnormalities are detected antenatally by ultrasound scan to allow proper care after birth.

FETAL TRAUMA

Fetal injuries can range from minor trauma, such as bruising or forceps marks, to major damage, such as fractures.

Procedure

- Inform the parents.
- Attend to the trauma if necessary.
- Discuss fully the likely cause and consequence of the trauma. Where appropriate offer an apology when the cause is clearly iatrogenic (e.g. skin incision to baby at caesarean section).
- Investigate fully where the cause is uncertain and inform the parents of the direction of the enquiry and its subsequent verdict.
- Document all proceedings in detail for medico-legal reasons.

FETAL DEATH

The stillbirth rate is around 5 per 1000 total births. Most (80%) stillbirths are unexplained fetal deaths where antepartum asphyxia is considered a direct cause (80%). In some 20% there may be a history of antepartum haemorrhage. Bleeding after 20 weeks and hypertensive disease remain as fetal risk factors.

Intrapartum asphyxia or trauma accounts for 10–15% of stillbirths. Failure to recognize a problem, inappropriate management and poor communication contribute to the adverse outcome.

Apart from the obvious disappointment facing all concerned, the response evoked in an individual can only be fully appreciated when the psychological background is considered. Medical personnel involved and a senior obstetrician should interview the couple jointly or on planned separate occasions. A tragedy such as this can greatly distress the staff as well as the couple concerned. Before counselling we must examine:

- our attitudes towards fetal loss
- our sense of guilt in terms of personal failure and the reasons why the obstetric system may have failed
- our ability to assess the aetiology objectively and identify avoidable factors
- our ability to detect pathological grief in the parents necessitating referral for psychiatric or social support
- our competency to conduct counselling.

Do not discourage discussion of the death or over-reassure and gloss over the tragedy. Too often clinicians have been viewed by parents as insensitive, unsympathetic and unconcerned. A suggested approach is as follows in Box 23.1.

Box 23.1 Stillbirth or fetal death protocol

- Confirm fetal death or stillbirth has occurred – inform the mother immediately.
- Allow ample time for both the mother and her partner to ventilate their feelings and seek causes.
- Do not make excuses. Adopt an accepting attitude. Guilt feelings in mothers are common. Expression of anger is therapeutic, allowing mothers to offload some of their guilt feelings.
- Remember fetal death or stillbirth may be viewed by the mother as further evidence of her failings and inadequacies. It can also be felt as the loss of part of herself and can stimulate fantasies analogous to that of phantom limbs after amputation. The birth of a child may hold symbolic significance as a means of

redeeming some of the mother's shortcomings in life. Search for these background factors in the discussion to understand the mother's responses and to assist in subsequent counselling. Existing children can be affected by the tragedy and may need help and counsel. Support for the couple must extend into the next pregnancy and next birth.

Management
- Confirm suspicion of fetal death by auscultation, cardiotocography and ultrasound scanning.
- Obtain detailed history. This may help determine the cause and is important for the management of subsequent pregnancies.

Box 23.1   *(Continued)*

- Take blood from the mother for haemoglobin, full blood count, cross-matching, clotting screen and Kleihauer count.
- Consider delivery. Mothers seldom wish to continue pregnancy once fetal death is confirmed. A quarter to a third may develop disseminated intravascular coagulation if the fetus is not delivered within 3–4 weeks.
- Transfusion or resuscitation may be necessary if fetal death followed placental separation. Problems with clotting may need to be corrected.
- Avoid caesarean section unless there are mechanical problems such as transverse lie. Aim for a delivery with minimum intervention, discomfort or surgical intervention.
- Allow labour to continue if contractions are present; otherwise if there is no contraindication induce labour at a time acceptable to the mother. The most effective method is the combination of the anti-progesterone agent mifepristone (600 mg) followed 36–48 hours later by oral or vaginal misoprostol (50 micrograms).
- Intravenous syntocinon can be used to augment labour.
- Leave membranes intact until labour is advanced (5 cm cervical dilatation) and delivery is assured. Prolonged rupture of membranes increases risk of intrauterine infection.
- Use analgesia (morphine or diamorphine) liberally. Discuss with the mother the degree of sedation she requires. An epidural block can be given provided there is no clotting defect.
- Keep delivery as uncomplicated as possible.

Following stillbirth
- Encourage the parents to see and hold the baby. If there is reluctance a photograph should be taken and kept for future reference. This practice will help identify the dead baby as an entity and facilitate parental mourning. The mother and father must be warned if there is gross abnormality or maceration. Display the baby to show as much normality as possible.
- Interview the couple on at least three occasions to provide opportunities for repeated discussion, to express empathy and to assess the couple's psychological status. Grief and the usual reactions to loss such as denial, guilt and aggression are normal responses but inappropriate behaviour indicates the need for psychiatric counselling.

Documentation
- Conduct detailed inspection for malformations, deformities, infection and trauma.
- Photograph abnormal or dysmorphic features.

- Skeletal radiography is mandatory to assist subsequent genetic counselling.
- Record occipitofrontal circumference, crown to heel length, limb length, etc.
- Conduct detailed inspection of the placenta, record weight, take swabs for culture and dispatch for pathological examination.
- At an appropriate time broach the sensitive question of post mortem or histology. Emphasize the value of this investigation to determine aetiology of fetal death and for subsequent care. If full autopsy is not allowed seek permission for limited biopsy of skin, lung and liver. Make sure the consent form is signed and full ethical details are on the request form (see Box 23.2).

Investigation
- Maternal blood should be screened for infection (TORCH, parvovirus, etc), Kleihauer count, liver and thyroid function, anti-cardiolipin antibodies and blood sugar.
- Take swabs from vagina, placenta and baby.
- Take fetal blood (cardiac puncture) for infection screen and examination of fetal chromosomes. Fetal skin (from the axilla so as not to disfigure) can be used for karyotyping (if no maceration, otherwise use muscle or cartilage).

Administration
- Inform as soon as possible all relevant persons such as GPs, community midwives, health visitors and other involved colleagues to avoid unnecessary or inadvertent comments. This will allow early arrangements for after care following discharge from hospital.
- Allocate a family room so the partner can stay. The baby, cleaned and dressed, is left with the couple to allow time to grieve in privacy. Notify religious advisor if this is requested.
- When gestation is more than 24 weeks a stillbirth certificate (issued by the obstetricians) and a certificate of burial or cremation (issued by a registrar of births and deaths) is required. Unless mothers request otherwise the law does not require burial or cremation for gestations before 24 weeks. If burial of the baby is intended, a certificate stating that the fetus was stillborn is required.
- In the UK a maternity grant allowance is payable for fetal death after 24 weeks.
- Mothers must all be given a postnatal follow-up appointment at the gynaecological clinic (away from an obstetric environment) to allow further discussion and counselling with the consultant obstetrician. Where appropriate refer for genetic counselling or psychiatric support.

Box 23.2   Post mortem request

- Consent for post mortem examination should be by a senior member of the obstetric team able to understand the sensitivity of the task; discuss reasons for the request; identify who performs the examination and where, and provide comprehensive information.
- Parents should know the value of the post mortem for identifying time and cause/causes of death: to confirm or elicit structural abnormalities and search for placental pathology.
- Information should include how the post mortem is performed (usually incision over back of the head to examine the brain and a midline neck to pelvis cut for access to relevant organs) and if organs (e.g. brain or heart) or tissues are likely to be retained.
- Consent for organ retention must be specifically

notated. This will include use for teaching, research or dispense for tests, e.g. metabolic and any additional consultation. If there is doubt consult the perinatal pathologist.
- Parents must be told when results are available and the length of time organs/tissues are retained (usually 3 weeks to 3 months).
- Where full post mortem is declined approach parents for a limited post mortem to answer specific questions or confirm diagnosis, e.g. heart lesion. In certain circumstances, e.g. metabolic disorders, tissue samples may need to be taken early.
- Parental consent is not needed for a coroner's autopsy.
- Fill in the structured post mortem request form. This will include a detailed history.

MATERNAL TRAUMA

Maternal trauma in the pelvic region can occur spontaneously during labour and delivery or as a consequence of operative delivery. Where possible minimize long term damage to urethral and anal sphincter.

Procedure

- Elicit the nature and the extent of damage.
- Explain and discuss any requirements for surgical repair and prognosis.
- If the cause is iatrogenic, offer an apology, explain the reason for the damage and adopt a neutral accepting role during any discussion.
- Document all proceedings fully for medico-legal reasons.

The medical profession is not taught to dispense harm or damage, but accidents can happen. An objective appraisal of the situation is instructive and experience gained can be used to benefit others. In current practice untoward incident forms must be completed for audit and action to avoid a recurrence.

MATERNAL DEATH

The death of any young person as a result of a natural function, which usually brings happiness, is a catastrophe. The fact that it occurs is a constant reminder of Nature's capriciousness, our need for further knowledge of obstetrics and, above all, a reminder that events may be difficult to predict and that constant vigilance is necessary in the care of our mothers.

Procedure

- The most senior person should inform, console and interview the husband/partner and relatives. Discuss fully all possible aetiologies.
- Notify the relevant staff and personnel, e.g. community midwives and GPs.
- Document fully all the proceedings for medico-legal reasons.
- Complete a death certificate.
- A post mortem is usually mandatory.
- A thorough investigation is always necessary.
- Adopt the same attitude as suggested for other misadventures during interviews.

FURTHER READING

Maternal and Child Health Consortium 2002 Confidential enquiry into stillbirths and deaths in infancy. Maternal and Child Health Consortium, London

Index